Current Trends in Neuropathology

Editor

DAVID M. MEREDITH

SURGICAL PATHOLOGY CLINICS

www.surgpath.theclinics.com

Consulting Editor
JASON L. HORNICK

June 2020 • Volume 13 • Number 2

ELSEVIER

1600 John F. Kennedy Boulevard • Suite 1800 • Philadelphia, Pennsylvania, 19103-2899

http://www.theclinics.com

SURGICAL PATHOLOGY CLINICS Volume 13, Number 2
June 2020 ISSN 1875-9181, ISBN-13: 978-0-323-75606-8

Editor: Katerina Heidhausen
Developmental Editor: Donald Mumford

Surgical Pathology Clinics (ISSN 1875-9181) is published quarterly by Elsevier Inc., 360 Park Avenue South, New York, NY 10010. Months of issue are March, June, September, and December. Business and Editorial Office: Elsevier Inc., 1600 John F. Kennedy Blvd., Ste. 1800, Philadelphia, PA 19103-2899. Accounting and Circulation Offices: Elsevier Inc., 3251 Riverport Lane, Maryland Heights, MO 63043. Periodicals postage paid at New York, NY and at additional mailing offices. Subscription prices are $219.00 per year (US individuals), $294.00 per year (US institutions), $100.00 per year (US students/residents), $272.00 per year (Canadian individuals), $335.00 per year (Canadian Institutions), $263.00 per year (foreign individuals), $335.00 per year (foreign institutions), and $120.00 per year (international students/residents), $100.00 per year (Canadian students/residents). Foreign air speed delivery is included in all *Clinics'* subscription prices. All prices are subject to change without notice. **POSTMASTER:** Send address changes to *Surgical Pathology Clinics*, Elsevier, 3251 Riverport Lane, Maryland Heights, MO 63043. **Customer Service: 1-800-654-2452 (US). From outside the United States, call 1-314-447-8871. Fax: 1-314-447-8029. E-mail:** JournalsCustomerServiceusa@elsevier.com **(for print support)** and JournalsOnlineSupport-usa@elsevier.com **(for online support).**

Reprints. For copies of 100 or more, of articles in this publication, please contact the Commercial Reprints Department, Elsevier Inc., 360 Park Avenue South, New York, NY 10010-1710. Tel. 212-633-3874; Fax: 212-633-3820; E-mail: reprints@elsevier.com.

Surgical Pathology Clinics of North America is covered in *MEDLINE/PubMed (Index Medicus).*

Contributors

CONSULTING EDITOR

JASON L. HORNICK, MD, PhD
Director of Surgical Pathology and
Immunohistochemistry, Brigham and Women's
Hospital, Professor of Pathology, Harvard
Medical School, Boston, Massachusetts, USA

EDITOR

DAVID M. MEREDITH, MD, PhD
Associate Pathologist, Department of
Pathology, Brigham and Women's Hospital,
Harvard Medical School, Boston,
Massachusetts, USA

AUTHORS

JARED AHRENDSEN, MD, PhD
Department of Pathology, Beth Israel
Deaconess Medical Center, Harvard Medical
School, Boston, Massachusetts, USA

SANDA ALEXANDRESCU, MD
Neuropathologist, Department of
Pathology, Boston Children's Hospital,
Assistant Professor of Pathology, Harvard
Medical School, Boston, Massachusetts, USA

WENYA LINDA BI, MD, PhD
Center for Skull Base and Pituitary Surgery,
Department of Neurosurgery, Brigham and
Women's Hospital, Harvard Medical School,
Boston, Massachusetts, USA

MELISSA M. BLESSING, DO
Clinical Fellow, Department of Pathology,
Boston Children's Hospital, Harvard Medical
School, Boston, Massachusetts, USA

JIE CHEN, MD, PhD
Assistant Professor, Department of Pathology
and Microbiology, University of Nebraska
Medical Center, Omaha, Nebraska, USA

SONIKA M. DAHIYA, MBBS, MD
Associate Professor, Department of
Pathology and Immunology, Washington
University School of Medicine, St. Louis,
Missouri, USA

PHEDIAS DIAMANDIS, MD, PhD
Laboratory Medicine Program, University
Health Network, Departments of Laboratory
Medicine and Pathobiology, and Medical
Biophysics, University of Toronto, Toronto,
Ontario, Canada

UGLJESA DJURIC, PhD
Laboratory Medicine Program,
University Health Network, Toronto,
Ontario, Canada

JOSEPH DRIVER, MD
Center for Skull Base and Pituitary Surgery,
Department of Neurosurgery, Brigham and
Women's Hospital, Harvard Medical School,
Boston, Massachusetts, USA

ADRIAN M. DUBUC, PhD, FACMG
Department of Pathology, Harvard Medical
School, Brigham and Women's Hospital,
Boston, Massachusetts, USA

KEVIN FAUST
Princess Margaret Cancer Centre, Department of Computer Science, University of Toronto, Toronto, Ontario, Canada

MEL B. FEANY, MD, PhD
Senior Pathologist, Department of Pathology, Brigham and Women's Hospital, Professor of Pathology, Harvard Medical School, Boston, Massachusetts, USA

JEFFREY HELGAGER, MD, PhD
Department of Pathology, Brigham and Women's Hospital, Harvard Medical School, Boston, Massachusetts, USA

SAMANTHA HOFFMAN, BS
Center for Skull Base and Pituitary Surgery, Department of Neurosurgery, Brigham and Women's Hospital, Harvard Medical School, Boston, Massachusetts, USA

MARY-JANE LIM-FAT, MD
Clinical Fellow, Center for Neuro-Oncology, Dana-Farber Cancer Institute, Boston, Massachusetts, USA

DAVID M. MEREDITH, MD, PhD
Associate Pathologist, Department of Pathology, Brigham and Women's Hospital, Harvard Medical School, Boston, Massachusetts, USA

LAKSHMI NAYAK, MD
Assistant Professor of Neurology, Center for Neuro-Oncology, Dana-Farber Cancer Institute, Boston, Massachusetts, USA

ADIL ROOHI, BSc
Harvard Extension School, Cambridge, Massachusetts, USA; Princess Margaret Cancer Centre, Toronto, Ontario, Canada

KATHERINE E. SCHWETYE, MD, PhD
Assistant Professor, Department of Pathology, Saint Louis University, St Louis, Missouri, USA

ISAAC H. SOLOMON, MD, PhD
Associate Pathologist, Department of Pathology, Brigham and Women's Hospital, Harvard Medical School, Boston, Massachusetts, USA

MATTHEW TORRE, MD
Postdoctoral Research Fellow, Department of Pathology, Brigham and Women's Hospital, Harvard Medical School, Boston, Massachusetts, USA

Contents

histology and associated molecular findings. Like elsewhere in brain biopsy evaluation, imaging is crucial and acts as a surrogate to gross examination. Given the circumscribed nature of these tumors, surgery alone is the mainstay treatment in most
entities.

Primary lymphoid neoplasms of the central nervous system are rare tumors that
span a wide range of histopathologic appearances and can overlap occasionally
with non-neoplastic processes. Application of modern molecular techniques has
not only begun to unravel their unique underlying biology but has also started to
lay a valuable diagnostic and therapeutic framework for these frequently aggressive
malignancies. This review summarizes the existing landscape of clinicopathologic
and genomic features of lymphoid neoplasms that may arise primarily within the
central nervous system.

Infections of the central nervous system cause significant morbidity and mortality in
immunocompetent and immunocompromised individuals. A wide variety of microorganisms can cause infections, including bacteria, mycobacteria, fungi, viruses, and
parasites. Although less invasive testing is preferred, surgical biopsy may be necessary to collect diagnostic tissue. Histologic findings, including special stains and
immunohistochemistry, can provide a morphologic diagnosis in many cases, which
can be further classified by molecular testing. Correlation of molecular, culture, and
other laboratory results with histologic findings is essential for an accurate diagnosis, and to minimize false positives from microbial contamination.

Mesenchymal tumors compromise an array of neoplasms that arise from or secondarily affect the central nervous system (CNS) and its surroundings. We review advances in understanding the molecular landscape of meningiomas and solitary
fibrous tumors, the most common primary CNS mesenchymal tumors. Molecular
findings most relevant to tumor diagnostics and prognostication are underscored.
As molecular techniques become more routinely incorporated into clinical practice,
such alterations may strengthen formal grading schemes and highlight novel therapeutic avenues.

Sellar region tumors include a broad range of benign and malignant neoplastic as well
as non-neoplastic entities, many of which are newly described or have recently revised
nomenclature. In contrast to other intracranial sites, imaging features in this region are
less specific, and the need for histopathological diagnosis is of paramount importance.
This review will describe pituitary adenomas, inflammatory lesions, and tumors unique
to the region (craniopharyngioma) as well as tumors which may occur in but are not
exclusively localized to the sellar location (schwannoma, metastasis, etc.).

Administration of systemic antineoplastic agents can result in adverse neurologic events. We describe the clinicopathologic features and putative mechanisms underlying iatrogenic neuropathology of the central nervous system secondary to chimeric antigen receptor (CAR) T-cell therapy and conventional chemotherapy.

Tumors of the central nervous system (CNS) have been historically classified according to their morphologic and immunohistochemical features. In 2016, updates to the classification of tumors of the CNS by the World Health Organization revolutionized this paradigm. For the first time, genomic findings, whether whole-arm chromosomal aberrations or single nucleotide variants, represent a necessary and critical component of diagnosis, contributing or superseding histologic findings. These updates stem from decades of technical innovation and genomic discovery. During this time, there has been a dramatic expansion and evolution in clinical genomic assays for these tumors, informing diagnosis and guiding therapeutic management.

Applications of artificial intelligence and particularly deep learning to aid pathologists in carrying out laborious and qualitative tasks in histopathologic image analysis have now become ubiquitous. We introduce and illustrate how unsupervised machine learning workflows can be deployed in existing pathology workflows to begin learning autonomously through exploration and without the need for extensive direction. Although still in its infancy, this type of machine learning, which more closely mirrors human intelligence, stands to add another exciting layer of innovation to computational pathology and accelerate the transition to autonomous pathologic tissue analysis.

SURGICAL PATHOLOGY CLINICS

SERIES OF RELATED INTEREST
Clinics in Laboratory Medicine

THE CLINICS ARE AVAILABLE ONLINE!
Access your subscription at:
www.theclinics.com

Preface
Current Trends in Neuropathology

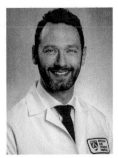

David M. Meredith, MD, PhD
Editor

The field of neuropathology has rapidly evolved over the past decade, largely due to the wealth of information generated by modern molecular technologies. The discovery of characteristic genomic alterations for a wide spectrum of neoplasms arising within the central nervous system has revolutionized the diagnostic approach to tumor classification, leading to the incorporation of widespread molecular definitions in the recent 2016 World Health Organization update. As our knowledge of tumor biology continues to grow, so will our need to carefully integrate new findings with traditional histopathologic evaluation.

This issue of *Surgical Pathology Clinics* covers several key areas where recent advances in molecular diagnostics are poised to impact current practice for pathologists and clinicians alike. For example, 3 articles are dedicated to pediatric brain tumors, which not only discuss updated genomic features of many existing neoplasms but also include newly described entities as well. Furthermore, molecular testing for mesenchymal neoplasms, lymphoid malignancies, and even infectious diseases is beginning to be utilized for diagnosis confirmation and treatment planning.

Beyond simply refining tumor classification schema, the age of molecular medicine ushers in new challenges and opportunities for the practicing neuropathologist. As the list of available tools continues to expand, understanding the ability and limitations of each assay can be challenging. To this end, a primer on the currently employed assays in brain tumor diagnosis is included in this issue. Because neuropathologists are being increasingly relied upon to perform and interpret genomic assays for treatment planning and trial enrollment, we have a unique opportunity to help design and participate in modern biomarker-based clinical trials; therefore, 1 article is dedicated to summarizing the current list of actionable events as well as general concepts of trial design.

These same advances in molecular diagnostics have been exploited clinically through the development of targeted agents and cellular therapies. Immunomodulation and the use of chimeric antigen receptor T cells are promising new treatment paradigms in oncology and are likely to be utilized with increasing frequency. Still, the off-target effects of these therapies are not well understood in the brain, but recent work demonstrates an expanding spectrum of iatrogenic neuropathology that will be

Surgical Pathology 13 (2020) ix–x
https://doi.org/10.1016/j.path.2020.03.001
1875-9181/20/© 2020 Published by Elsevier Inc.

critical to recognize as we examine the efficacy of novel agents and which is summarized herein.

Finally, we must consider what will likely be the next revolution in our field: applying artificial intelligence to image analysis. Currently, available deep learning algorithms have made great strides at being able to accurately recognize diverse tissue elements and histologic diagnoses, and a discussion of the capabilities and limitations of this technology is included in this issue.

This diverse collection of articles aims to serve not only as an update for several rapidly evolving areas of neuropathology but also as a reference for integrating molecular diagnostics into clinical practice.

David M. Meredith, MD, PhD
Department of Pathology
Brigham and Women's Hospital
75 Francis Street
Boston, MA 02115, USA

E-mail address:
dmmeredith@bwh.harvard.edu

Genomic Biomarker Assessment in Gliomas
Impacts of Molecular Testing on Clinical Practice and Trial Design

Mary-Jane Lim-Fat, MD[a], Lakshmi Nayak, MD[a,1],
David M. Meredith, MD, PhD[b,*,1]

KEYWORDS

• Glioma • Biomarker • Clinical trial • Genomic

Key points

- Recently revised classification schema for gliomas issued by the World Health Organization and the Consortium to Inform Molecular and Practical Approaches to CNS Tumor Taxonomy integrate numerous genomic biomarkers that facilitate more accurate diagnosis and assessment of prognosis, and oncologists increasingly rely on molecular testing results for treatment planning.

- The wealth of genomic data for gliomas has facilitated the development of numerous clinical trials exploring the efficacy of targeted and immunomodulatory agents, necessitating routine molecular testing for these tumors.

- Given the genomic heterogeneity of gliomas and the narrow window of time for treatment planning, turn-around-time and cost-effectiveness of comprehensive biomarker assessment continue to pose major challenges for personalized treatment.

ABSTRACT

Recent discoveries elucidating the genetic underpinnings of glial neoplasms have revealed myriad recurrent alterations that have clinical value by improving accuracy of diagnosis and prognosis. Furthermore, this wealth of genomic information provides the basis for targeted therapies and the subsequent design of biomarker-based clinical trials. This review summarizes the current landscape of clinically relevant molecular alterations in gliomas and describes the role of routine molecular testing in context of treatment planning for standards of care and clinical trials.

OVERVIEW

Concerted efforts to characterize chromosomal abnormalities, genomic mutations, epigenomic alterations, and proteomic changes have provided a deeper knowledge and appreciation of the biology and taxonomy of brain tumors. In 2016, a revision to the World Health Organization (WHO) classification of central nervous system (CNS) tumors highlighted the integration of molecular diagnostics to complement histologic diagnosis and grading.[1] This has now been incorporated in practice guidelines, endorsed by the National Comprehensive Cancer Network (NCCN) and the Consortium to Inform Molecular and Practical Approaches to CNS Tumor Taxonomy (cIMPACT-NOW).[2]

---

[a] Center for Neuro-Oncology, Dana Farber Cancer Institute, 450 Brookline Ave, Boston, MA 02215, USA;
[b] Department of Pathology, Brigham and Women's Hospital, Harvard Medical School, 75 Francis Street, Boston, MA 02115, USA
[1] Contributed equally.
* Corresponding author.
E-mail address: dmmeredith@bwh.harvard.edu

Surgical Pathology 13 (2020) 209–215
https://doi.org/10.1016/j.path.2020.02.003
1875-9181/20/© 2020 Elsevier Inc. All rights reserved.

Across many glioma types, copy number alterations, mutational events, and gene rearrangements, as well as tumor mutational burden and methylation profiles have been described and can help broaden our understanding of each tumor's distinct natural history, vulnerabilities, response, and progression patterns. Although many of these changes are yet to be incorporated into widespread clinical practice and in some instances require further validation, these unprecedented advances hold great promise in improving early diagnosis, identifying prognostic and predictive patterns, and finding the best treatment for each patient.

In this review, we discuss how the latest updates in genomic signatures promise to revolutionize care for patients with glioma by helping to inform diagnosis, treatment selection, and prognosis prediction.

CURRENT INTEGRATION OF GENOMICS IN CLINICAL PRACTICE: DIAGNOSIS AND PROGNOSIS

The classification of brain tumors over the past decade has undergone a major paradigm shift with the advent of more widespread use of molecular diagnostic techniques. Next-generation sequencing (NGS), in combination with chromosomal arrays and fusion assays, has allowed for more precise regrouping of gliomas of similar biological lineages and behavior, moving toward integrated histologic/molecular diagnoses with more rigorous diagnostic reproducibility.

MOLECULAR DIAGNOSIS IN ADULT DIFFUSE GLIOMAS

New understanding of the molecular changes driving gliomagenesis was at the basis for the 2016 revision to the WHO CNS tumor classification schema and has proven to be of significant prognostic relevance in glioma. Most important in diffuse adult gliomas are isocitrate dehydrogenase (IDH) mutations and 1p/19q co-deletion status. IDH-mutant diffuse gliomas are further separated into astrocytomas and oligodendrogliomas, depending on whether they possess co-occurring ATRX and TP53 mutations or 1p/19q co-deletion, respectively. Given the mutual exclusivity of these events, the histologic diagnosis of oligoastrocytoma has no molecular equivalent and has thus been abandoned.[1] In addition, a provisional framework allowing for the molecular diagnosis of glioblastoma can now be made in IDH-wild-type astrocytic tumors in which an EGFR amplification, TERT promoter mutation, or chromosome 7 gain or 10 loss is identified, regardless of their histologic grade.[3]

A specific and accurate tissue diagnosis is central to the initial patient-provider discussion and establishes the plan of care and prognosis discussion. Specifically, with regard to treatment, the approach to high-grade gliomas routinely includes a gross total resection, followed by adjuvant chemoradiation and adjuvant chemotherapy with temozolomide, an alkylating agent.[4] In low-grade gliomas, although practice may vary depending on the patient's age, extent of resection, size of the tumor, and provider preferences, a combination of resection, radiation, and chemotherapy with temozolomide or with a combination of procarbazine, lomustine (CCNU), and vincristine (collectively referred to as PCV) is typically prescribed.[5]

The power of ancillary molecular testing to refine and correct histologic diagnoses (especially in the setting of surgical undersampling) was quickly recognized, leading to the development of consensus guidelines for integrated diagnosis reporting.[6] As a result, many current clinical trials have specific inclusion criteria pertaining to the integrated diagnosis, granting many more patients access to cutting edge therapies. As more and more patients are enrolled into clinical trials requiring biomarker assessment via molecular testing, the importance of timely integrated diagnostic reporting becomes even greater. This process can be limited by a number of factors, including access to surgical expertise, size of tumor sample, and availability of pathologic expertise and molecular testing.

PROGNOSTIC AND PREDICTIVE MARKERS IN GLIOMAS

An important cornerstone of clinical care of patients with brain tumor relies on an understanding of prognosis and predicting tumor response to therapy. This is particularly important in a vulnerable patient population in which, in addition to prolonging survival, maximizing quality of life and limiting potentially harmful treatments is a primary consideration.

As discussed previously, IDH1/2 mutations have become central to the classification of diffuse gliomas and has helped stratify prognosis across all histologic grades. In IDH-mutant Grade III astrocytomas, the median overall survival is approximately 10 years, whereas in IDH-mutant Grade IV glioblastoma, the overall survival is approximately twice that of their IDH-wild-type counterpart.[7] However, even within the Grade II and Grade III IDH-mutant diffuse astrocytomas, somatic copy number alterations, in particular homozygous deletions of CDKN2A/B, also have been found to be associated with a more aggressive course, prompting a novel grading of diffuse gliomas.[8]

Methylation at the promoter region of the O6-methylguanylmethyltransferase (MGMT) gene in patients with newly diagnosed glioblastoma has been found to be a strong predictive marker in terms of response to alkylating therapy or radiotherapy. Based on the Stupp trial published in 2005, the median overall survival with concurrent chemoradiation and adjuvant therapy with temozolomide for MGMT-methylated patients with glioblastoma was 23.4 months, whereas it was only 12.6 months in the MGMT-unmethylated group.[9] With more robust validation of MGMT methylation, replacing temozolomide by investigational agents through a clinical trial in unmethylated glioblastoma has become a reasonable option, particularly as the NCCN guidelines now endorse offering clinical trials to both patients with newly diagnosed glioblastoma and those with recurrent eligible glioblastoma. In MGMT-methylated newly diagnosed patients, there has also been interest in capitalizing on a combination of 2 alkylating nitrosureas, and a recently published study investigated the combination of lomustine-temozolomide compared with standard of care therapy in the concurrent radiation and adjuvant stage. The combination group had an overall survival of 48.1 months compared with 31.4 in the temozolomide-alone group.[10] However, potential additive myelosuppressive effects may limit this strategy.

In patients older than 65 years, concurrent fractionated radiation therapy and temozolomide remains the first choice of treatment.[11] Nonetheless, in patients who otherwise have poorer functional status, several studies support the use of temozolomide alone in MGMT-methylated patients and conversely the use of radiation therapy alone in MGMT-unmethylated patients.[12,13] The significance of MGMT methylation in lower-grade gliomas remains less clear, as these tumors retain both MGMT alleles (found on chromosome 10q) in contrast to glioblastomas.[14] However, as testing becomes more widely available, correlation with patient outcomes may provide more insight into its predictive or prognostic capability in low-grade gliomas or other tumors.

Adult and pediatric diffuse midline gliomas harboring mutations in histone variants H3.1 (HIST1H3B) or H3.3 (H3F3A) at the K27 codon have been recognized as a unique entity, as highlighted by the 2016 revision to the WHO classification.[1] H3K27M tumors can occur in both adult and pediatric patients, and the mutation is mutually exclusive with IDH1/2 mutation and is rarely found to have MGMT promoter methylation.[15,16] Because of their behavior, these tumors have been assigned a Grade IV diagnosis, irrespective of their histologic features, given that these tumors are often found in a difficult location, and biopsies are typically preferred. Detection of this mutation has been very helpful in opening clinical trial and therapeutic avenues by supporting the diagnosis of a highly aggressive tumor. In pediatric high-grade gliomas harboring this mutation, the overall survival is approximately 2.3 years shorter,[17] and survival in adults is equivalent to other IDH-wild-type gliomas.[16]

HYPERMUTATION IN GLIOMAS

Hypermutated gliomas, whether arising from germline defects in mismatch repair enzymes or acquired secondary to prior treatment with temozolomide, have been the subject of great interest, especially in the era of immunotherapy. Available tumor sequencing panels now have the capability of determining the tumor mutational burden, although the exact cutoff determining "hypermutation" has not been clearly established. In other systemic tumors with microsatellite instability and high mutational burden, such as colorectal cancer, immune checkpoint blockade has been associated with significant and sustained response.[18] However, immunogenicity of CNS tumors, in particular gliomas that acquire hypermutation secondary to temozolomide exposure, has not been well described. Clinical trials investigating PD-1 checkpoint blockade with pembrolizumab in pediatric patients with constitutional mismatch repair deficiency syndrome (ClinicalTrials.gov Identifier: NCT02359565), as well as in adults with recurrent glioblastomas with hypermutator phenotype (ClinicalTrials.gov Identifier: NCT02658279), are currently ongoing to determine the potential benefit of immune checkpoint blockade in these tumors.

TARGETED THERAPIES IN GLIOMAS

Despite our unprecedented understanding of gliomas and their genetic lineage, efforts to find effective therapies have fallen short. This is related to several different challenges, including the redundancy of several oncogenic pathways, lack of CNS penetrance from tested therapies, and intratumoral and intertumoral heterogeneity. Despite these obstacles, targeted therapies, based on individualized tumor genotyping and phenotyping, continue to hold great promise, aided by a better understanding of drivers of gliomagenesis.

In glioblastoma, several different targets have been identified. *EGFR* amplification occurs in approximately 50% of glioblastoma. Although prior small molecule inhibitors of *EGFRvIII* variant have failed to show significant benefit in clinical trials, a new antibody-drug conjugate targeting amplified *EGFR*, depatuxizumab mafodotin (ABT-414), delivers the active compound monomethyl auristatin F directly into cells harboring mutant *EGFRvIII*, thus circumventing classic EGFR inhibition and cell resistance.[19] A placebo-controlled Phase 2 b/3 study of radiotherapy/temozolomide against radiotherapy/temozolomide in combination with ABT-414 (RTOG 3508- ClinicalTrials.gov Identifier: NCT02573324) has been completed, with promising interim analysis data, although final results are expected in the coming year.

Targeted therapies for *BRAF* alterations have now been well-established in malignant melanoma. Although only approximately 1% to 2% of adult glioblastomas harbor a $BRAF^{v600E}$ mutation,[20] the accessibility of new inhibiting agents offers an attractive treatment option for this subgroup of patients. An open-label multicenter phase 2 basket study in patients with $BRAF^{v600E}$ rare cancers of several histologic types (Clinical-Trials.gov Identifier: NCT02034110) contained a subgroup of patients with high-grade glioma who received a combination of dabrafenib (*BRAF*-inhibitor) and trametinib (*MEK*-inhibitor). This study is currently ongoing, although interim individual patient data analysis has indicated sustained response in some participants. Of note, targeted therapy with *BRAF* inhibitors also has been used in other nonglial CNS tumors. In craniopharyngiomas, NGS has helped differentiate between papillary craniopharyngiomas, which contain the $BRAF^{v600E}$ mutation, and adamantinomatous craniopharyngiomas, which contain the exon 3 activating *CTNNB1* mutations.[21] Targeted therapy with *BRAF* inhibitors for papillary craniopharyngiomas is being investigated and has shown optimistic results in many cases.[22]

Multikinase inhibitors, such as regorafenib, which targets vascular endothelial growth factor receptor, angiopoietin 2, platelet-derived growth factor receptor, and fibroblast growth factor receptor, also have been investigated recently in glioblastoma, having had a longer track record in other systemic cancers. The REGOMA (Regorafenib in Relapsed Glioblastoma) trial enrolled patients with recurrent glioblastoma and randomized salvage therapy with lomustine against regorafenib. Median overall survival in the regorafenib group was 7.4 versus 5.6 months in the lomustine-treated group.[23] Clinical trials using the CNS penetrant dopamine receptor D2 antagonist (DRD2) ONC201 (ClinicalTrials.gov Identifier: NCT02525692) are currently ongoing after a phase 2 study showed some antitumoral activity in a patient with recurrent *H3K27M*-mutant glioblastoma. Other targeted therapies are currently being investigated, including panobinostat, a general histone deacetylase inhibitor with in vitro efficacy against *H3K27M*-mutant diffuse pontine gliomas.[24] Other targets currently being investigated in gliomas include CDK4/6 (abemaciclib, ribociclib, palbociclib), *NTRK* fusion (larotrectinib, entrectinib), and *MDM2* amplification (AMG232).

IDH1 and IDH2 play a crucial role in converting isocitrate to α-ketoglutarate. Mutations in *IDH1* or *IDH2* lead to an overproduction of 2-hydroxyglutarate (2-HG), which has been revealed to be an oncometabolite in several tumor types and a compelling therapeutic target.[25] A number of *IDH1* (eg, AG120, IDH305, AGI5198), *IDH2* (AGI6780, AG221), and combined inhibitors (AG-881) are therefore in various stages of clinical testing. More broadly, this enzymatic pathway offers several other potential targets, including glutaminase inhibitors and the potential to combine *IDH*-inhibitors with vaccines or checkpoint inhibitors due to effective immune-modulation by 2-HG in glioma.[26] The latter strategy is being explored in a currently active study of PD-1 inhibition in recurrent or progressive *IDH*-mutant gliomas (ClinicalTrials.gov Identifier: NCT03557359).

USE OF BIOMARKERS IN CLINICAL TRIALS AND RESPONSE ASSESSMENT

The current landscape of clinical trials in gliomas does not represent an effective means to test out potential treatment targets, as the median time to completion of clinical trials in glioblastoma is 3 to 4 years.[27] Newer and innovative clinical trial designs aim to address this issue, a prominent example of which is the Individualized Screening Trial of Innovative Glioblastoma Therapy (INSIGhT) trial (ClinicalTrials.gov Identifier: NCT02977780), a Bayesian adaptive platform trial for patients with newly diagnosed glioblastoma with a 2-phase approach.[28] In this design, randomization at diagnosis occurs to multiple experimental arms or one control arm, and patient subtypes, including biomarkers, are identified, after which adaptive randomization occurs based on accumulating trial results. Based on interim results, arms can be dropped while new arms can be added over time. On a global scale, GBM AGILE (Glioblastoma adaptive, global, innovative learning environment) aims to use a similar platform for patients with recurrent glioblastoma with accrual set to begin in the coming year.[29]

Endpoints and response assessment in brain tumors in the context of clinical trials pose a particular challenge in the context of intertumoral heterogeneity, as well as temporal and spatial intratumoral heterogeneity. RNA sequencing provides posttranscriptional data reflecting more accurate changes in tumor cell biology and also promises to offer more insight into individual tumor response and mechanism of resistance. However, this is currently time intensive and costly and has not been fully implemented in the clinical world. Posttreatment or midtreatment data on tumor samples is also limited by the fact that tissue analysis would require invasive sampling. Although neoadjuvant trials, in which the investigative agent is administered before tissue sampling and analysis have been a paradigm shift, temporal sampling across the disease and treatment spans capturing new mutations is not always feasible.

Sampling and sequencing of cell-free circulating tumor DNA (ctDNA) in plasma or blood has been considered as a possible mechanism to circumvent the need of multiple repeat craniotomies for tissue analysis. In particular, sequencing of ctDNA from cerebrospinal fluid (CSF) has yielded longitudinal data on brain tumors, paralleling the changes in tumor burden, and characterizing biomarkers more accurately than in plasma ctDNA.[30] The genomic landscape of gliomas was further characterized in 42 of a cohort of 85 patients with glioma, in which tumor-derived DNA was detected in CSF.[31] Concordance between the CSF ctDNA genomic profile and that of the tumor biopsy was demonstrated, and alterations reflecting temporal evolution in the tumor DNA was also captured in CSF. CSF ctDNA may therefore represent a less invasive method to assess for new targetable mutations throughout the evolution of brain tumors.

PRACTICAL CONSIDERATIONS AND COST-EFFECTIVENESS

As larger validated reference datasets emerge for specific tumor types, curated and relevant NGS assays have become available for gliomas. These platforms can be institution dependent (SNaPshot, OncoPanel, or GlioSeq) or commercially available (FoundationOne CDx) and can contain several hundreds of selected genes. Individual analysis of gliomas for mutations that are potentially targetable has been integrated in several workflows and is particularly crucial for enrollment in clinical trials that may have specific mutations as inclusion criteria. It is also increasingly helping to shape clinical practice with the increased availability of "off-label" drug repurposing for targetable mutations.

The cost of sequencing with newer NGS panels can nonetheless be daunting, and extensive molecular genotyping in the absence of clear targetable mutations and effective therapies may not represent a cost-effective strategy. New studies using cost-modeling analyses are therefore helping clarify financially effective testing algorithms. For example, an algorithm to identify EGFR-amplified, IDH-wild-type lower-grade diffuse gliomas was developed with the understanding that accurate diagnosis in this particular population has important clinical ramifications but does not necessarily entail extensive and costly sequencing.[32] As understanding of relevant targets and drivers of oncogenesis becomes clearer, cost-effectiveness analyses may help identify other combined strategies that can best help patients on an individual level.

Another concern is whether molecular testing is feasible in the timeline of real-world best clinical practice. Although some groups have been able to integrate a workflow of 5 days from tissue biopsy to finalized report of a 130 NGS gene panel,[33] in most institutions, this can take several weeks and presents a challenge in glioblastoma where a treatment plan needs to be formulated within 2 to 4 weeks from the date of surgery. In addition, with the increase in number of trials for newly diagnosed glioblastomas, molecular information, including MGMT status, is typically needed within 2 weeks after surgery at initial consultation with the neuro-oncologist before radiation planning.

As cost-effective and efficient NGS technology becomes more widely available, a vast amount of molecular data will need to be analyzed, correlated, and validated to create a more comprehensive repository of relevant changes and their impact on patients. Managing and sharing these datasets to be able to deduct meaningful conclusions will pose several challenges from an infrastructure and cost standpoint. A collaborative effort from scientists, clinicians, and software engineers will be required to translate big data into precision medicine to ultimately help patients who need better treatments.

DISCLOSURE

The authors have no sources of funding to disclose. The authors declare no conflict of interest.

REFERENCES

1. Louis DN, Perry A, Reifenberger G, et al. The 2016 World Health Organization classification of tumors of the central nervous system: a summary. Acta Neuropathol 2016;131(6):803–20.
2. Louis DN, Aldape K, Brat DJ, et al. cIMPACT-NOW (the consortium to inform molecular and practical approaches to CNS tumor taxonomy): a new initiative in advancing nervous system tumor classification. Brain Pathol 2017;27(6):851–2.
3. Brat DJ, Aldape K, Colman H, et al. cIMPACT-NOW update 3: recommended diagnostic criteria for "Diffuse astrocytic glioma, IDH-wildtype, with molecular features of glioblastoma, WHO grade IV". Acta Neuropathol 2018;136(5):805–10.
4. Stupp R, Mason WP, van den Bent MJ, et al. Radiotherapy plus concomitant and adjuvant temozolomide for glioblastoma. N Engl J Med 2005;352(10): 987–96.
5. Brown TJ, Bota DA, van Den Bent MJ, et al. Management of low-grade glioma: a systematic review and meta-analysis. Neurooncol Pract 2019;6(4): 249–58.
6. Louis DN, Perry A, Burger P, et al. International Society of Neuropathology–Haarlem consensus guidelines for nervous system tumor classification and grading. Brain Pathol 2014;24(5):429–35.
7. Cancer Genome Atlas Research Network, Brat DJ, Verhaak RG, Aldape KD, et al. Comprehensive, integrative genomic analysis of diffuse lower-grade gliomas. N Engl J Med 2015;372(26):2481–98.
8. Shirahata M, Ono T, Stichel D, et al. Novel, improved grading system(s) for IDH-mutant astrocytic gliomas. Acta Neuropathol 2018;136(1):153–66.
9. Hegi ME, Diserens AC, Gorlia T, et al. MGMT gene silencing and benefit from temozolomide in glioblastoma. N Engl J Med 2005;352(10):997–1003.
10. Herrlinger U, Tzaridis T, Mack F, et al. Lomustine-temozolomide combination therapy versus standard temozolomide therapy in patients with newly diagnosed glioblastoma with methylated MGMT promoter (CeTeG/NOA-09): a randomised, open-label, phase 3 trial. Lancet 2019;393(10172):678–88.
11. Perry JR, Laperriere N, O'Callaghan CJ, et al. Short-course radiation plus temozolomide in elderly patients with glioblastoma. N Engl J Med 2017; 376(11):1027–37.
12. Wick W, Platten M, Meisner C, et al. Temozolomide chemotherapy alone versus radiotherapy alone for malignant astrocytoma in the elderly: the NOA-08 randomised, phase 3 trial. Lancet Oncol 2012; 13(7):707–15.
13. Malmstrom A, Gronberg BH, Marosi C, et al. Temozolomide versus standard 6-week radiotherapy versus hypofractionated radiotherapy in patients older than 60 years with glioblastoma: the Nordic randomised, phase 3 trial. Lancet Oncol 2012; 13(9):916–26.
14. Hartmann C, Hentschel B, Tatagiba M, et al. Molecular markers in low-grade gliomas: predictive or prognostic? Clin Cancer Res 2011;17(13):4588–99.
15. Solomon DA, Wood MD, Tihan T, et al. Diffuse midline gliomas with histone H3-K27M mutation: a series of 47 cases assessing the spectrum of morphologic variation and associated genetic alterations. Brain Pathol 2016;26(5):569–80.
16. Meyronet D, Esteban-Mader M, Bonnet C, et al. Characteristics of H3 K27M-mutant gliomas in adults. Neuro Oncol 2017;19(8):1127–34.
17. Lu VM, Alvi MA, McDonald KL, et al. Impact of the H3K27M mutation on survival in pediatric high-grade glioma: a systematic review and meta-analysis. J Neurosurg Pediatr 2018;23(3):308–16.
18. Colle R, Cohen R, Cochereau D, et al. Immunotherapy and patients treated for cancer with microsatellite instability. Bull Cancer 2017;104(1):42–51.
19. van den Bent M, Gan HK, Lassman AB, et al. Efficacy of depatuxizumab mafodotin (ABT-414) monotherapy in patients with EGFR-amplified, recurrent glioblastoma: results from a multi-center, international study. Cancer Chemother Pharmacol 2017; 80(6):1209–17.
20. Schindler G, Capper D, Meyer J, et al. Analysis of BRAF V600E mutation in 1,320 nervous system tumors reveals high mutation frequencies in pleomorphic xanthoastrocytoma, ganglioglioma and extra-cerebellar pilocytic astrocytoma. Acta Neuropathol 2011;121(3):397–405.
21. Brastianos PK, Taylor-Weiner A, Manley PE, et al. Exome sequencing identifies BRAF mutations in papillary craniopharyngiomas. Nat Genet 2014; 46(2):161–5.
22. Brastianos PK, Shankar GM, Gill CM, et al. Dramatic response of BRAF V600E mutant papillary craniopharyngioma to targeted therapy. J Natl Cancer Inst 2016;108(2).
23. Lombardi G, De Salvo GL, Brandes AA, et al. Regorafenib compared with lomustine in patients with relapsed glioblastoma (REGOMA): a multicentre, open-label, randomised, controlled, phase 2 trial. Lancet Oncol 2019;20(1):110–9.
24. Grasso CS, Tang Y, Truffaux N, et al. Functionally defined therapeutic targets in diffuse intrinsic pontine glioma. Nat Med 2015;21(7):827.
25. Dang L, Su SM. Isocitrate dehydrogenase mutation and (R)-2-hydroxyglutarate: from basic discovery to therapeutics development. Annu Rev Biochem 2017;86:305–31.
26. Pellegatta S, Valletta L, Corbetta C, et al. Effective immuno-targeting of the IDH1 mutation R132H in a murine model of intracranial glioma. Acta Neuropathol Commun 2015;3:4.

27. Vanderbeek AM, Rahman R, Fell G, et al. The clinical trials landscape for glioblastoma: is it adequate to develop new treatments? Neuro Oncol 2018;20(8): 1034–43.

28. Alexander BM, Trippa L, Gaffe S, et al. Individualized screening trial of innovative glioblastoma therapy (INSIGhT): a Bayesian adaptive platform trial to develop precision medicines for patients with glioblastoma. JCO Precis Oncol 2019;(3):1–13.

29. Alexander BM, Ba S, Berger MS, et al. Adaptive global innovative learning environment for glioblastoma: GBM AGILE. Clin Cancer Res 2018;24(4): 737–43.

30. De Mattos-Arruda L, Mayor R, Ng CKY, et al. Cerebrospinal fluid-derived circulating tumour DNA better represents the genomic alterations of brain tumours than plasma. Nat Commun 2015;6:8839.

31. Miller AM, Shah RH, Pentsova EI, et al. Tracking tumour evolution in glioma through liquid biopsies of cerebrospinal fluid. Nature 2019;565(7741): 654–8.

32. Bale TA, Jordan JT, Rapalino O, et al. Financially effective test algorithm to identify an aggressive, EGFR-amplified variant of IDH-wildtype, lower-grade diffuse glioma. Neuro Oncol 2019;21(5):596–605.

33. Sahm F, Schrimpf D, Jones DT, et al. Next-generation sequencing in routine brain tumor diagnostics enables an integrated diagnosis and identifies actionable targets. Acta Neuropathol 2016;131(6): 903–10.

An Update on Pediatric Gliomas

Jared Ahrendsen, MD, PhD[a], Sanda Alexandrescu, MD[b],*

KEYWORDS

• Pediatric glioma • NTRK • EWSR1 • FGFR • HGNET-BCOR • BCOR-EP300

Key points

- Although the histology of pediatric gliomas can be indistinguishable from adult gliomas, their biology is distinct and it informs the diagnosis and prognosis.
- Gliomas with novel class-defining genetic events are emerging and can pose diagnostic challenges.
- Co-occurring genetic events in pediatric gliomas can be helpful in establishing a specific diagnosis and in guiding clinical management.

ABSTRACT

Pediatric gliomas are biologically distinct from adult gliomas. Although recent literature uncovered new genetic alterations, the prognostic implications of these discoveries are still unclear. This article provides an update on the histologic and molecular features with prognostic and/or therapeutic implications in pediatric gliomas.

purposes, most tumors that are classified by the World Health Organization (WHO) as grade I or II are discussed as low-grade gliomas, whereas tumors that are WHO histologic grade III or IV are generally discussed as high-grade gliomas. This article does not discuss the recent progress made in glioneuronal tumors, because that is the subject of a separate article in this issue.

OVERVIEW

Brain tumors are currently the leading cause of cancer-related death in pediatric patients.[1,2] Among them, low-grade gliomas are the most common (approximately 30% of all brain tumors) and are associated with significant morbidity, whereas high-grade gliomas are rare but incurable with currently available therapies.[3] Both low-grade and high-grade pediatric gliomas are clinically and biologically distinct from adult gliomas[4] and there is not enough published guidance regarding their histologic grading, specific classification, and outcomes.

This article covers the recent diagnostic, genetic, and prognostic discoveries in low-grade and high-grade pediatric gliomas. For practical

PEDIATRIC LOW-GRADE GLIOMAS

Pediatric low-grade gliomas (PLGGs) are the most common brain tumors in children, representing 30% of all central nervous system (CNS) tumors. Despite their low mortality, they represent a significant challenge because of their high morbidity and multiple recurrences. PLGGs are clinically and biologically distinct from adult low-grade gliomas. The adult diffuse gliomas are characterized by *IDH* mutations, but these mutations are rare in children; almost all PLGGs are driven by genetic alterations that influence mitogen-activated protein kinase (MAPK) signaling pathway, and, among those, *BRAF* alterations are the most common.[5] This article reviews pilocytic astrocytoma, pilomyxoid astrocytoma, angiocentric glioma, pleomorphic xanthoastrocytoma, and emerging

[a] Department of Pathology, Beth Israel Deaconess Medical Center, Harvard Medical School, 330 Brookline Ave, Boston, MA 02115, USA; [b] Department of Pathology, Boston Children's Hospital, Harvard Medical School, 300 Longwood Avenue, Bader 104, Boston, MA 02115, USA
* Corresponding author.
E-mail address: Sanda.Alexandrescu@childrens.harvard.edu

Surgical Pathology 13 (2020) 217–233
https://doi.org/10.1016/j.path.2020.02.005

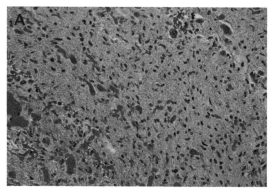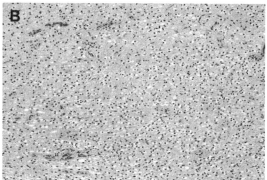

Fig. 1. PA. (A) PAs are composed of cells with round to oval mildly atypical nuclei and with piloid processes. Rosenthal fibers are frequent. (B) PAs sometimes show oligodendrogliomalike features.

entities with characteristic histology and molecular results.

PILOCYTIC ASTROCYTOMA

Among PLGGs, pilocytic astrocytoma (PA) is the most common and it represents 5.4% of all pediatric and adult gliomas.[2] It can occur anywhere along the neuraxis, but has a predilection for posterior fossa and, more specifically, cerebellum. Radiologically, PA appears as a well-demarcated solid and cystic tumor with contrast enhancement. On histology, PAs are composed of bipolar, mildly atypical cells with oval nuclei (Fig. 1A). They are usually biphasic tumors, with more cellular areas alternating with foci that are less cellular and have a myxoid background. Focal oligodendrocytelike morphology is common (Fig. 1B). Rosenthal fibers and eosinophilic granular bodies are usually present, and pseudocysts bordered by linear microvascular proliferation are common; in the setting of a PA, the microvascular proliferation should not prompt a concern for high-grade glioma. Occasionally, PAs have a mild or moderately high mitotic rate and proliferation index,[3] which is an accepted feature and not concerning for a higher-grade lesion.

Most PAs have activation of MAPK signaling through numerous alterations, of which the most common is a tandem duplication at 7q34 that results in *KIAA1549-BRAF* fusion, which is found in 98% of the posterior fossa cases.[6] The *BRAF* duplication can be observed through fluorescence in situ hybridization, array comparative genomic hybridization, or fusion assays. Although *BRAF* tandem duplication remains the most common event independent of location, more recent studies described numerous other genetic alterations that result in MAPK pathway activation: *BRAF V600E* mutation, *BRAF* intragenic deletions and insertions, *NTRK* fusions, and *FGFR1* and *KRAS* point mutations.[7–9]

PA is the CNS neoplasm most frequently associated with neurofibromatosis type 1 (NF1); in that setting, the most common location is the optic pathway.[10] Although NF1 is inherited in an autosomal-dominant pattern, approximately two-thirds of the cases of NF1 are caused by a sporadic mutation in the *NF1* gene encoding neurofibromin. Patients with NF1 have only 1 functional *NF1* gene. The second hit seen in PAs associated with NF1 syndrome occurs through point mutations or loss of heterozygosity.

Rarely, PA can be a symptom of Noonan syndrome, which is caused by germline mutations in MAPK pathway genes, the most common being *PTPN11*.[11]

The prognosis of PA is very good, with more than 95% of the patients being alive 5 to 10 years after surgical resection.[12] Histologic grade is usually maintained, and only rare cases develop anaplastic histology, usually after radiation or chemotherapy. Location and ability to resect the entire tumor are key factors in prognosis.[13]

PILOMYXOID ASTROCYTOMA

Pilomyxoid astrocytoma (PMA) affects mostly infants and young children, with a median age of 10 months. The most common location is the hypothalamus/optic pathway, although PMAs can be encountered anywhere in the neuraxis. The tumor was previously considered a distinct entity with a histologic WHO grade II, because of a possible less favorable prognosis than PA. Recent research showed that PMA and PA have similar biological backgrounds[14]; therefore, the 2016 WHO classification of the CNS tumors describes it as a histologic variant of PA and without a grade assigned. On histology, PMA has a pronounced myxoid background in which cells are arranged in a stellate, angiocentric fashion. Unlike PA, PMA lacks Rosenthal fibers and eosinophilic granular bodies. The literature hypothesizes that their more aggressive behavior is caused by the young age at presentation and tumor location, which often makes a complete resection impossible.

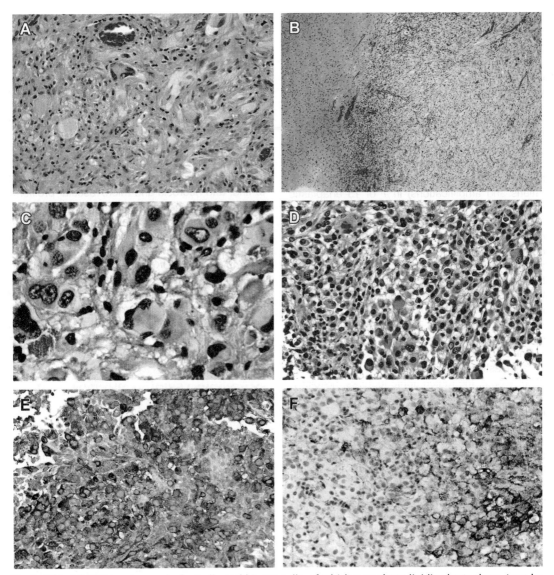

Fig. 2. PXA. (*A*) PXA is composed of spindle and bizarre cells, of which some have lipidized cytoplasm. Lymphocytes can be present around the vessels and admixed with the tumor (hematoxylin-eosin [H&E]). (*B*) Usually there is a sharp demarcation between PXA and surrounding brain (H&E). (*C*) Eosinophilic granular bodies are a common finding in PXA, and the periodic acid–Schiff (PAS) special stain can highlight them (PAS). (*D*) An example of epithelioid PXA composed of cells with abundant eosinophilic cytoplasm, eccentric nuclei, prominent nucleoli, and distinct cellular borders (H&E). (*E*) BRAF V600E immunostain is positive in most PXAs. (*F*) Epithelioid PXAs show patchy epithelial membrane antigen (EMA) immunoexpression.

PLEOMORPHIC XANTHOASTROCYTOMA

Pleomorphic xanthoastrocytoma (PXA) is a solid, noninfiltrative, epileptogenic tumor of childhood and young adulthood. It usually occurs in the superficial temporal lobe, involving the cortex, superficial white matter, and sometimes leptomeninges; however, it can occur anywhere in the CNS. On histology, PXA is composed of glial cells with spindled morphology admixed with bizarre, sometimes multinucleated, cells (**Fig.** 2A, B). Xanthomatous changes and scattered eosinophilic granular bodies are common (**Fig.** 2C), and the tumor creates a characteristic reticulin-rich network around individual cells (not shown). Although PXA is regarded as a WHO grade II tumor with good prognosis after complete surgical resection, occasional cases have increased mitotic rate (4 or more per 10 high-power fields) and necrosis, prompting a WHO grade III classification. Sometimes anaplastic PXAs can have epithelioid morphology, making it difficult to distinguish from epithelioid glioblastomas (**Fig.** 2D). In such instances, focal features of classic PXA that include eosinophilic granular bodies indicate an anaplastic PXA.

Approximately 50% to 78% of PXAs have *BRAF* point mutations, the most common being *BRAF V600E* immunostain is used in clinical practice as a surrogate for the specific mutation (**Fig.** 2E).[15] Another common alteration in PXA is loss of chromosome 9, encountered in 50% of the cases.[16] Homozygous deletion of *CDKN2A/2B* is present in 60% of PXAs. A recent study by Phillips and colleagues[17] showed *TERT* alterations (hotspot mutations and amplifications) in 7 of 15 anaplastic PXAs included in the cohort.

The diagnosis of PXA can be challenging, especially when the histology is anaplastic or the tumor does not harbor a *BRAF V600E* mutation. In such situations, in order to distinguish these cases from other gliomas and particularly from glioblastoma, comprehensive molecular characterization is needed. Phillips and colleagues[18] described *ATG7-RAF1* and *NRF1-BRAF* fusions in 2 cases of anaplastic PXA without *BRAF V600E*.

One of the challenges in practice is differentiating an anaplastic epithelioid PXA from an epithelioid glioblastoma; the radiographic features, histology, and molecular background of these tumors are often indistinguishable. Both are solid tumors composed of large cells with abundant cytoplasm and nuclei with prominent nucleoli. Like PXA, epithelioid glioblastoma tends to have a superficial location and to involve leptomeninges.[19] They both have BRAF V600E mutations and, interestingly, focal EMA immunopositivity (**Fig.** 2F). A recent study by Korshunov and colleagues[20] showed that epithelioid glioblastomas stratify into established diagnostic categories on clustering methylome analysis, with a subset of pediatric glioblastomas clustering with PXAs and having a good prognosis.

ANGIOCENTRIC GLIOMA

Angiocentric glioma was first described in 2005 by Wang and colleagues[21] as an infiltrative low-grade epileptogenic cerebral glioma showing T2 hyperintensity on MRI. The tumors are composed of bipolar cells with elongated nuclei, which infiltrate the brain matter and show angiocentricity (**Fig.** 3). Glial immunomarkers are positive. Mitoses are difficult to find, and necrosis and microvascular proliferation are usually not encountered. In the study by Wang and colleagues,[21] all but 1 patient were free of disease after surgical resection, with a follow-up ranging from days to 62 months. Recently, a *MYB-QKI* gene fusion was identified as the defining genetic alteration in most angiocentric gliomas.[22] The 2016 WHO definition of angiocentric glioma is a grade I cerebral tumor; however, in 2017, 3 almost simultaneous articles described angiocentric gliomas arising in the brainstem, challenging the WHO definition.[23-25]

LOW-GRADE PEDIATRIC GLIOMAS WITH NEWLY DISCOVERED MOLECULAR ALTERATION

Diffuse low-grade gliomas in the pediatric population are difficult to classify in a specific category; they challenge the WHO grading system, which is primarily applicable to adult diffuse gliomas.[3] Pediatric diffuse low-grade gliomas are usually negative for *IDH*, *ATRX*, and *p53* mutations, and usually do not have 1p/19q whole arm codeletion. Application of comprehensive clinical molecular studies leads

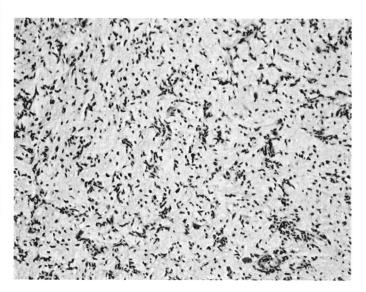

Fig. 3. Angiocentric glioma. Angiocentric glioma is an infiltrative low-grade epileptogenic neoplasm with elongated, mildly atypical cells that display angiocentric arrangement in a myxoid background stroma.

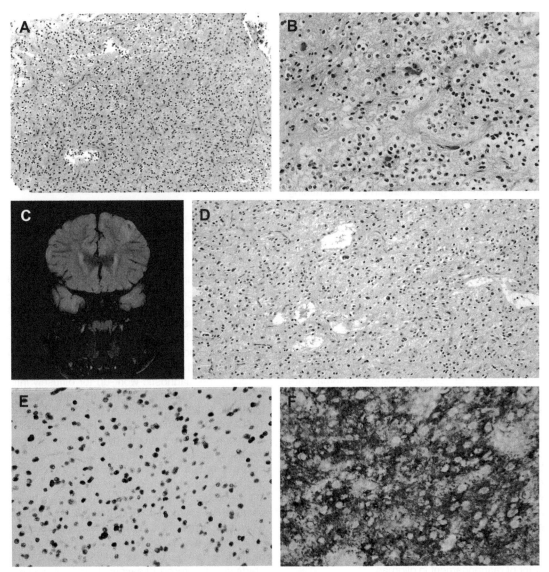

Fig. 4. (*A, B*) A diffuse pediatric glioma with *FGFR3-TACC3* rearrangement; it is composed of oligodendrocytelike cells with round and oval nuclei, perinuclear clearing, and occasional delicate vessels (H&E). (*C–F*) A polymorphous low-grade neuroepithelial tumor of youth with *FGFR2-CTNNB1* rearrangement in a 17-year-old patient. (*C*) T2 fluid-attenuated inversion recovery MRI showing an infiltrative superficial tumor in the left frontal lobe. (*D*) The glioma is composed of cells with mild-to-moderate nuclear atypia, occasional microcysts and delicate vascular channels (H&E). (*E*) OLIG2 immunostain is diffusely expressed and (*F*) the tumor cells are positive for EMA immunoexpression. Mitoses, microvascular proliferation, and necrosis are absent.

to the discovery of diffuse low-grade gliomas with *FGFR* point mutations and fusions,[26] *NTRK* fusions,[27] as well as more rare fusions involving unexpected genes, such as *EWSR1* and *BCOR*.[28,29]

Aside from PA with *FGFR* point mutations (mostly p.N546K and p.K656E), *FGFR1* point mutations and *FGFR* fusions can be present in a subset of pediatric diffuse gliomas in any location in the neuraxis. The most common fusions are *FGFR1-TACC1*, *FGFR2-CTTNA3*, and *FGFR3-TACC3* fusions. Another common *FGFR* alteration in pediatric

gliomas is *FGFR1 TKD*. In one of the authors' experience (S.A.), *FGFR1-TACC1* and *FGFR3-TACC3* fusions can be seen in both low-grade and high-grade diffuse pediatric gliomas (**Fig. 4**A, B).

In the authors' experience, gliomas with *FGFR2-CTTNA3* fusions have common clinical, radiologic, histologic, and molecular features. Patients usually present with seizures and a hemispheric mass (**Fig. 4**C); microscopic examination shows an infiltrative glial neoplasm with cells with speckled chromatin and perinuclear clearing (oligolike features), a rich network of delicate vascular channels, and scattered calcifications (**Fig. 4**D). The tumor cells are diffusely positive for glial markers (**Fig. 4**E) and sometimes they can show diffuse CD34 immunopositivity (**Fig. 4**F), similar to the tumors described by Huse and colleagues[30] as polymorphous low-grade neuroepithelial tumor of the young (PLNTY). In this study of 10 tumors diagnosed as PLNTY with a follow-up ranging from 12 to 89 months, a single patient had new seizures and progression 36 months after gross total resection; the rest of the patients were without evidence of disease after surgical management, resembling the clinical course of a WHO grade I glioma. The tumors that did not have *FGFR2-CTNNA3* fusion had *BRAF V600E* mutation, or *FGFR2-KIAA1549* fusions; they all had a similar behavior.

Alterations in tropomyosin-related kinase (TRK) genes are found mostly in adult and infantile glioblastomas.[31,32] The authors have encountered in practice pediatric diffuse gliomas with *NTRK* rearrangements of all grades; their histology seems to vary from case to case and there seems to be no correlation between histology and a particular *NTRK* gene or fusion partner, although specific studies on larger cohorts of *NTRK*-rearranged gliomas are needed for meaningful conclusions. In order to show the range of histologic features of *NTRK*-rearranged gliomas, 2 cases, 1 with low-grade and 1 with high-grade histology, are shown in **Fig. 5**. At present, there are no well-defined studies describing the outcome of patients with *NTRK*-fused gliomas. Although the use of pan-TRK antibody is becoming widespread in mesenchymal tumors, its use in neuropathology practice needs to take into consideration that normal brain expresses TRK proteins and positivity is expected in normal circumstances, hence the immunosurrogate is not an objective indicator of rearrangement in gliomas.

With the increased number of molecular modalities, fusions between *EWSR1* and novel partners have been described in soft tissue tumors. Alterations in *EWSR1* were not described in gliomas until 2019, when Siegfried and colleagues[28] reported a case of an intraventricular glioneuronal tumor with *EWSR1-PATZ1* fusion (exon 8 of *EWSR1* and exon 1 of *PATZ1*). The histology of the described tumor is low grade with areas of increased cellularity, pleomorphism, and a rich network of hyalinized vessels. The tumor is positive for OLIG2, and focally positive for glial fibrillary acidic protein (GFAP) and synaptophysin. Methylation analysis indicated that the tumor is distinct from all other well-described entities. In addition, 3 large-scale sequencing studies on pediatric and adult gliomas contain 3 gliomas with *EWSR1-PATZ1* fusion, of which 1 is described as high grade.[33–35] However, these studies do not comment on histology and outcomes and do not speculate on whether these tumors represent a new entity or not. The senior author of this article (S.A.) encountered a case of an intraventricular glioma with an *EWSR1-PATZ1* fusion (**Fig. 6**). The histology was similar to that described by Siegfried and colleagues[28] for case 1: the tumor had increased cellularity and pleomorphism and a rich vascular network, but it lacked microvascular proliferation, mitoses were rare, and there was no necrosis, prompting a diagnosis of low-grade glioma. Unlike Siegfried and colleagues'[28] case, this case did not have neuronal features.

GLIOMAS WITH ISOCITRATE DEHYDROGENASE MUTATIONS IN PEDIATRIC PATIENTS

The WHO groups diffuse infiltrating gliomas based on the presence or absence of isocitrate dehydrogenase (*IDH*) mutations, with *IDH*-mutated tumors in either diffuse astrocytoma (which have co-occurring *TP53* and *ATRX* mutations) or oligodendroglioma (defined by the presence of *IDH* mutation and 1p/19q whole arm codeletion) categories. In practice, the diagnostic work-up for diffusely infiltrating gliomas involves (1) immunohistochemistry for IDH1 R132H, p53, and ATRX; (2) analysis of 1p/19q status by fluorescent in situ hybridization, array comparative genomic hybridization, or polymerase chain reaction; and, if available, (3) targeted next-generation sequencing to identify molecular oncogenic driver mutations and fusions.[36]

Low-grade infiltrating gliomas in adults are nearly ubiquitously driven by *IDH1* or *IDH2* mutations,[3] whereas *IDH* mutations are exceedingly uncommon in low-grade gliomas of childhood. A landmark study profiling whole-genome sequencing of 151 low-grade gliomas from 149 patients found only a single *IDH*-mutated tumor in a 15-year-old patient.[37] Ferris and colleagues[38] describe a short series of 3 young patients (9, 9, and 7 years old) with diffuse astrocytomas with IDH mutations. This study shows the possible presence of IDH mutations in children younger than 10 years; interestingly, 2 of the patients in this series had intact ATRX expression and lacked *ATRX* and *TERT* promoter mutations, suggesting that some *IDH*-mutant gliomas in children might be distinct from their adult counterpart.

The youngest patient with an *IDH1*-mutant diffuse astrocytoma seen at our institution was a 6-year-old patient with a frontal lobe glioma; histologically, the tumor was indistinguishable from an adult-type diffuse glioma WHO grade II (**Fig. 7**) and targeted exome sequencing confirmed the *IDH1(R132H)* mutation, but did not reveal any *ATRX*, *TP53*, *TERT* mutations or 1p/19q whole

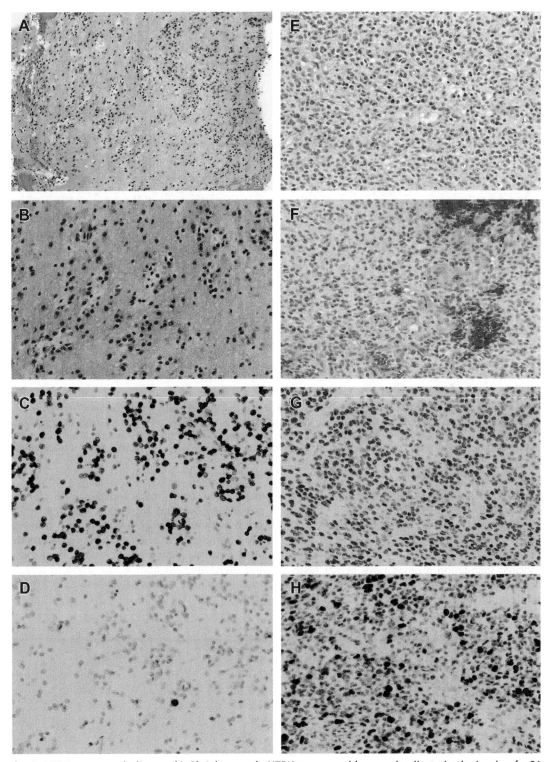

Fig. 5. NTRK-rearranged gliomas. (*A–D*) A low-grade NTRK-rearranged low-grade glioma in the insula of a 21-year-old patient. (*A*) The infiltrative glioma is arranged in hypercellular nests admixed with areas that are less cellular (H&E). (*B*) The cells have oligodendrocytelike features and mild nuclear atypia. No mitoses, necrosis, or microvascular proliferation were seen (H&E). (*C*) OLIG2 immunostain was diffusely positive and (*D*) the Ki67 proliferation-labeling index was 1% to 2%. (*E–H*) An NTRK-rearranged high-grade glioma in the parietal lobe of a 4-year-old patient. (*E, F*) show a densely cellular neoplasm composed of cells with oval, moderately atypical nuclei. Occasional mitoses are present, and foci containing microvascular proliferation were easily identified (H&E).

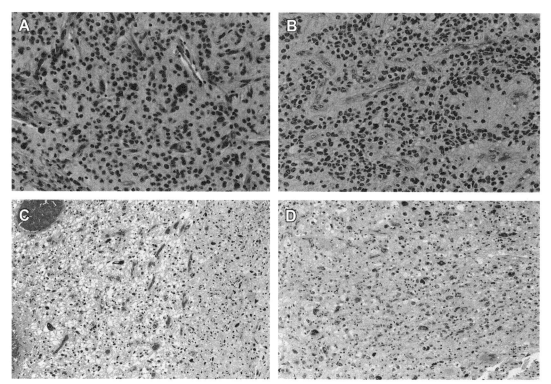

Fig. 6. Glioma with *EWSR1-PATZ1* rearrangement. The histology of this case was highly variable, with oligoden-drocytelike areas and a rich network of delicate vessels (*A*) admixed with areas in which the cells were monoto-nous and had a vague pseudorosette pattern (*B*). Some foci resembled low-grade glioneuronal tumors with a myxoid background stroma, spindled-appearing cells, some with nuclear atypia (*C*) and scattered ganglionlike cells (*D*).

arm codeletion. This case supports the conclusion in Ferris and colleagues[38] study.

PEDIATRIC HIGH-GRADE GLIOMAS

Pediatric high-grade gliomas have similar histo-logic features to their adult counterparts, but they are biologically different. In recent years there have been major advances in genetic profiling of pediatric high-grade gliomas, which led to separation of some entities from histolog-ically similar adult and pediatric counterparts. Most pediatric high-grade gliomas are primary, and transformation from a low-grade to a high-grade glioma is estimated at less than 10% in children.[38]

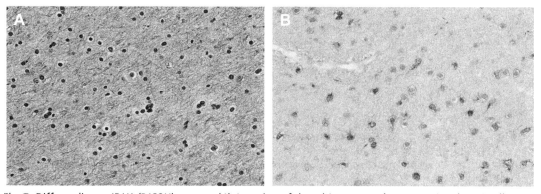

Fig. 7. Diffuse glioma, *IDH1 (R132H)* mutant. (*A*) A section of the white matter shows occasional minimally atyp-ical nuclei; overall the histology is similar to that of a mildly reactive white matter. (*B*) An IDH1 immunostain high-lights all the mutant cells.

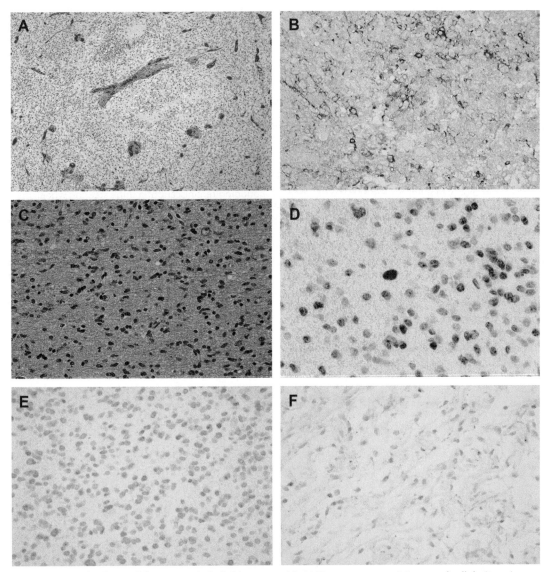

Fig. 8. High-grade glioma. (*A*) A congenital glioblastoma with *ALK1* rearrangement: increased cellularity, microvascular proliferation, and necrosis are present. (*B*) ALK1 immunostain shows significant positivity. (*C*) Representative diffuse midline glioma with occasional mitoses. (*D*) H3K27M immunostain shows crisp nuclear staining in most tumor cells, in keeping with *H3K27M* mutation; this patient was confirmed to have an *H3F3A* mutation. (*E*) Pale nuclear H3K27M immunostaining that was observed in a diffuse midline glioma with confirmed *HIST1H3B* mutation. (*F*) Granular cytoplasmic staining in some of the cells in a midline glioma confirmed negative for histone H3 mutations.

CONGENITAL AND INFANTILE HIGH-GRADE GLIOMAS

Among pediatric high-grade gliomas, congenital and infantile glioblastomas are sometimes biologically distinct from those occurring beyond this age. Congenital high-grade gliomas are often detected at prenatal ultrasonography as an echogenic, usually hemispheric large mass that produces midline shift and hydrocephalus. Genetically, these tumors are distinct from high-grade glioma in childhood and adulthood and

they tend to have better outcomes; although they can harbor loss of *PTEN* and *TP53* mutations, *EGFR* amplification, *IDH*, and histone mutations have not been described.[39] Recent publications and clinical observations show enriched *MET/ALK/ROS1/NTRK* alterations in a subset of congenital and infantile high-grade gliomas.[31,34] This discovery is particularly important for management, because *ALK1* inhibitors are used in some adult malignancies and experimental studies on glioblastoma lines exist.[40] **Fig. 8**A, B shows an *ALK*-rearranged congenital glioblastoma.

Beyond infancy, alterations in histone H3 (most commonly *H3F3A*, *HIST1H3B*, and *G34V/R*), *BRAF*, *NTRK*, and *BCOR* are known oncogenic drivers in pediatric diffuse high-grade gliomas.

HISTONE H3-MUTATED GLIOMAS

Diffusely infiltrating tumors arising in midline structures often harbor *H3K27M* mutations, and this group of tumors is associated with aggressive biological activity and poor clinical outcome.[41,42] This group includes most diffuse intrinsic pontine gliomas (DIPGs), many midline glioblastomas, and a small proportion of histologically low-grade diffuse astrocytomas located in midline structures.[37,43] As a result, in 2016, these tumors became recognized as a distinct grade IV entity by current WHO guidelines (diffuse midline glioma, K3K27M mutant, WHO grade IV) regardless of their histologic appearance.[3] A classic case of a diffuse midline glioma with H3K27M mutation and the patterns of expression of the H3K27M antibody are shown in **Fig. 8**C–F.

Pediatric midline gliomas harbor mutually exclusive mutations in 1 of 2 genes: the histone H3.3 gene *H3F3A* or H3.1 *HIST1H3B*.[44] The *H3K27M* mutations are primarily found in midline gliomas arising in the brainstem, spinal cord, and thalamus, although Zhang and colleagues[37] observed 1 case of low-grade diffuse astrocytoma with *H3K27M* mutation located in the cerebral hemisphere. Distinct histologic features and differences in clinical outcome between brainstem tumors with *H3.3K27M* and *H3.1K27M* have been described, with worse prognosis in the *H3.3K27M* group.[45]

In contrast, G34V/R mutations of *H3F3A* occur almost exclusively in hemispheric pediatric high-grade gliomas, and patients experience better overall survival.[46] Again, there are notable differences in clinical and molecular characteristics between K27M and G34R/V mutation, suggesting that these tumors have unique oncogenic derivation and likely represent distinct diseases.[47]

H3K27M mutations are not specific to diffuse gliomas, and have been identified in posterior fossa ependymoma,[48,49] PA,[50,51] and ganglioglioma.[52] The authors have encountered 1 such case of a ganglioglioma with *BRAF V600E* and *H3K27M* mutation located in the cervical spine of a 7-year-old patient who presented with excoriation disorder and asymmetric forearm muscle bulk (**Fig. 9**). Pages and colleagues[52] reported 5

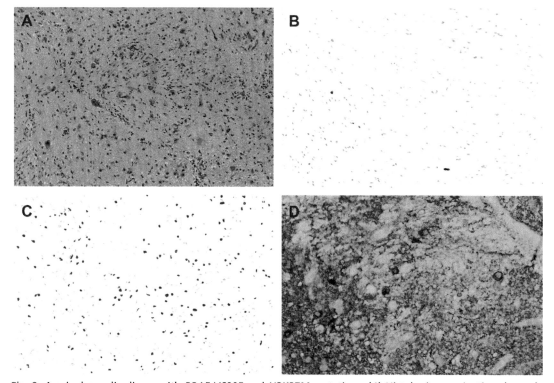

Fig. 9. A spinal ganglioglioma with *BRAF V600E* and *H3K27M* mutations. (*A*) Histologic examination showed a mildly cellular neoplasm composed of atypical glial cells admixed with clusters of large, disorganized neurons with dysplastic features (H&E). (*B*) The Ki67 immunostain showed a proliferation rate of approximately 1%. (*C*) The H3K27M immunostain was positive in the glial component and (*D*) BRAF V600E was positive in both glial and neuronal components.

similar midline pediatric gangliogliomas at WHO grade I (2 thalamic, 1 in the pons, 1 spinal, and 1 in the cerebellar penduncle) with co-occurring mutations in BRAF V600E and H3K27M. Of the 5 patients reported, 4 had follow-up, of which 3 were alive with stable disease at 9 months, 1 year, and 7 years, and 1 died of recurrent disease at 8 years. This series suggests that not all H3K27M-mutated gliomas should be graded as WHO IV. H3K27M mutations can also co-occur with FGFR1 point mutations; however, the outcome implication of this association is not fully described.[53] Given the existent short series and case reports on such cases, the Consortium to Inform Molecular and Practical Approaches to CNS Tumor Taxonomy Now Working Committee 3 released clarifying diagnostic criteria suggesting that the diagnosis of diffuse midline glioma, H3K27M mutant, WHO grade IV should be reserved for those gliomas that are diffusely infiltrating, in a midline location, and harboring an H3K27M mutation.[54] Given that many PAs and gangliogliomas show areas of infiltration and can occur in midline locations, it is possible that these guidelines can still allow for challenges in diagnosis. In challenging diagnoses, analyzing the co-occurring genetic events of an H3K27M-mutant glioma is useful, because the WHO grade IV gliomas typically have alterations in PDGFRA, ACVR1, ATRX, and TP53.[45]

Bona fide diffuse midline gliomas with H3K27M mutations have a 2-year overall survival of less than 10%.[3] Factors associated with longer survival include younger age, longer symptom latency, and absent ring enhancement on MRI.[55] A large study of more than 1000 patients with radiographically confirmed DIPG showed additional prognostic information, including that H3.1 K27M is associated with longer survival than H3.3 K27M.[56]

Of practical significance, although the availability of a mutation-specific H3K27M antibody facilitates the diagnosis,[57] awareness of limitations should be observed. First, the H3K27M antibody detects mutations associated with more than just a single gene. In our experience, dark nuclear staining is more associated with H3F3A mutation, whereas lighter, more speckled staining pattern is associated with HIST1H3B mutation. Furthermore, staining should only be interpreted as positive when observed in tumor nuclei (not cytoplasmic expression) and in the context of appropriate positive and negative controls (see Fig. 8). In addition, although H3K27M-mutant tumors are associated with loss of H3K27me3 expression, the latter is not specific for H3K27M mutation and should not be used as a surrogate for the mutation-specific antibody.[58]

BRAF V600E MUTATION IN HIGH-GRADE GLIOMAS

The most common BRAF alteration encountered in high-grade gliomas is BRAF V600E. Mistry and colleagues,[59] in a study of 886 patients with pediatric low-grade glioma, analyzed 26 cases that progressed to secondary high-grade gliomas. The most common alteration in secondary high-grade gliomas was BRAF V600E and CDKN2A loss, and all high-grade gliomas harboring these alterations could be traced back to their low-grade counterparts, although the transformation was of long duration. High-grade gliomas with BRAF V600E mutation tended to also have TP53 mutations. It was concluded that BRAF V600E mutations and CDKN2A deletions constitute a clinically distinct subtype of high-grade glioma. None of the high-grade gliomas in this cohort from Sick Kids Hospital had KIAA1549-BRAF fusion. Given the available targeted therapeutic options in clinical trials, it is important to determine whether a glioma harbors BRAF alterations and the type of alteration. Clinical trials usually include strata for BRAF V600E–mutant tumors and for without them, because BRAF V600E inhibitors can paradoxically activate the MAPK pathway through ERK signaling in BRAF-fused gliomas.[60] The BRAF V600E immunohistochemical stain is a good tool to screen for mutation; however, its interpretation can be uncertain and molecular confirmation through digital droplet polymerase chair reaction or a targeted sequencing panel that includes the BRAF gene is more sensitive.

NTRK REARRANGEMENTS IN HIGH-GRADE GLIOMAS

NTRK fusions can be seen in both low-grade and high-grade gliomas,[31,33] and their morphology is variable. In our clinical experience, it is difficult to assign a histologic grade to a subset of gliomas with NTRK rearrangement because their histology does not fit perfectly in any of the conventional entities. A case encountered in practice shows this (Fig. 10): a 3-year-old child presented with a brief history of headaches, and imaging showed a third ventricular well-defined tumor with an area of infiltration in the midbrain. A biopsy was performed and it showed a minimally infiltrative tumor composed of back-to-back monomorphic cells with round to oval nuclei and abundant eosinophilic cytoplasm. Occasional mitoses were seen, but there was no microvascular proliferation or necrosis. Eosinophilic granular bodies and Rosenthal fibers were not present. The tumor was diffusely positive for GFAP and

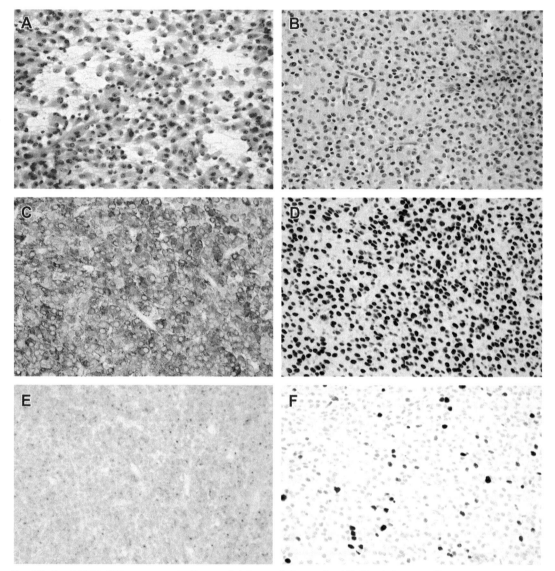

Fig. 10. An *NTRK3-EV6*–rearranged glioma of intermediate grade. (*A*) The intraoperative smear preparation showed a monomorphic population of cells with eccentric nuclei and abundant eosinophilic cytoplasm. Definitive processes were not seen (H&E). (*B*) The paraffin-embedded H&E section showed a tumor composed of monomorphic epithelioid cells with sheetlike pattern of growth as well as occasional papillaelike structures. (*C*) The GFAP and (*D*) OLIG2 immunostains were diffusely positive, in keeping with a glioma. (*E*) Synaptophysin was expressed in a cytoplasmic and dotlike pattern. (*F*) The Ki67 immunostain shows areas of moderately increased proliferation. There was no necrosis and no microvascular proliferation.

OLIG2 and also showed some patchy synaptophysin expression. The Ki67 was focally increased to 7%. Given the presence of occasional mitoses in a small biopsy, by WHO grading scheme, there was concern for a grade III tumor; however, the tumor appeared monomorphic and mostly noninfiltrative. Therefore, a diagnosis of glioma with some concerning features was rendered and the child was placed on low-grade glioma therapy. A fusion panel showed an *NTRK3-ETV6* fusion. More than a year after the

diagnosis, the tumor grew approximately 3 mm, which is atypical for a high-grade glioma, and the patient was placed on targeted therapy.

High-grade gliomas with *NTRK* fusions have all the histologic characteristics of glioblastoma.

Given the new progress in targeted therapy, uncovering *NTRK* rearrangements in pediatric gliomas is important for patient care. Because TRK proteins are expressed in the normal brain, panTRK immunostain is not a good immunosurrogate for gliomas, hence fluorescence in situ hybridization or a fusion panel is more appropriate whenever a *NTRK*-rearranged glioma is suspected.

NEW HIGH-GRADE GLIOMA ENTITIES

In 2016, Sturm and colleagues[60] performed comprehensive genomic and methylation characterization of 323 tumors diagnosed as primary CNS-PNETs at multiple collaborating institutions. The study showed that most of the tumors clustered with known entities, and there were 4 new entities with distinct histology and biology: CNS neuroblastoma with *FOXR2* activation (CNS NB-*FOXR2*), CNS Ewing sarcoma family tumor with *CIC* alteration (CNS EFT-*CIC*), CNS high-grade neuroepithelial tumor with *MN1* alteration (CNS HGNET-*MN1*), and CNS high-grade neuroepithelial tumor with *BCOR* alteration (CNS HGNET-*BCOR*). Of these, tumors from the CNS HGNET-*MN1* and CNS HGNET-*BCOR* entities expressed GFAP, whereas neuronal immunomarkers were positive only focally or were negative. Most tumors in the CNS HGNET-*MN1* category were well circumscribed and high grade, and contained a mixture of solid and pseudopapillary patterns, some resembling astroblastoma. Because most of the tumors histologically diagnosed as astroblastoma were in this category, it was considered unlikely that there is a true astroblastoma entity other than the *MN1*-altered tumors found by this study.

The CNS HGNET-*BCOR* consisted of relatively well-defined tumors with glial features composed of spindle and oval cells arranged in perivascular pseudorosettes. The *BCOR* alteration found in these tumors is a tandem duplication in exon 15, which is the same alteration described in clear cell sarcomas of kidney. **Fig. 11** shows the histology of such a case encountered in our clinical practice. Recently, Torre and colleagues[29] described 3 gliomas with *BCOR-EP300* fusion and distinct morphology that clustered together and separately from any other entities, including CNS HGNET-*BCOR*, on methylation clustering analysis, indicating that they represent a specific entity. This discovery also suggests that a more specific nomenclature for CNS HGNET-*BCOR* is needed. All 3 tumors in this study were large supratentorial gliomas with a myxoid/microcystic background stroma; frequent calcifications, including psammomatous; and prominent chicken-wire vessels. All 3 cases had areas of low-grade morphology and 2 of them also showed areas of anaplasia, potentially suggesting progression from a low-grade to a high-grade lesion. Representative photographs of such a case are shown in **Fig. 12**. BCOR immunohistochemical stain is a reliable surrogate for *BCOR* gene alterations in gliomas and it is positive in both HGNET-*BCOR* ITDex15 and in *BCOR-EP300* gliomas (see **Fig. 12**).

RADIATION-INDUCED HIGH-GRADE GLIOMAS

Among pediatric high-grade gliomas, the tumors that are secondary to prior radiotherapy should be mentioned. Radiotherapy improves survival of many pediatric cancers, but one of the side effects is increased risk of radiation-induced malignancy. Gliomas can arise after cranial or craniospinal radiation; almost all of them are high-grade and have particularly unfavorable outcome. In a series of 12 radiation-induced gliomas described by Lopez and colleagues,[61] 10 were high grade; of those, 7 harbored *TP53* mutations. The second most common genetic alteration was homozygous deletion of *CDKN2A* and *CDKN2B*. Other alterations encountered were *PDGFRA* and *MET* amplification, and *BRAF* and

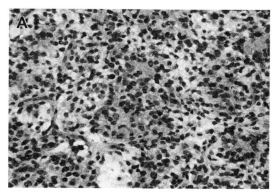
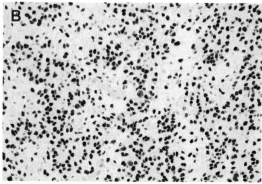

Fig. 11. HGNET-BCOR ITDex15 (*A*) Glioma composed of cells with round to oval atypical nuclei with vague perivascular arrangement around delicate vessels. Mitotic and apoptotic figures were easily found. (*B*) Nuclear BCOR immunostains were present in all tumor cells.

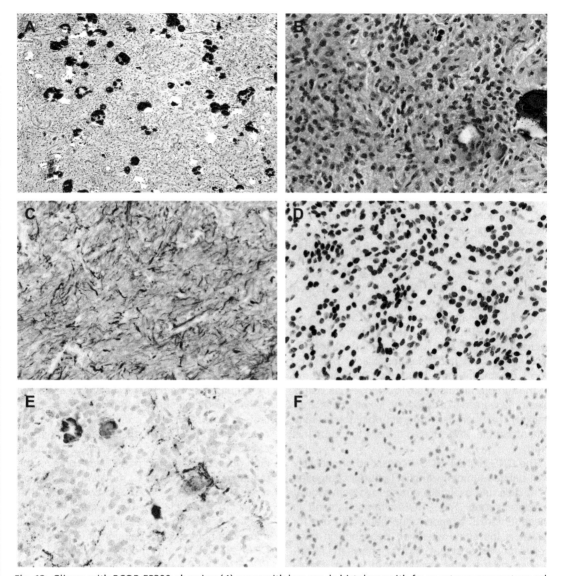

Fig. 12. Glioma with BCOR-EP300, showing (*A*) areas with low-grade histology with frequent psammomatous calcifications; moderate cellularity; mild atypia; and a network of thin, delicate vessels (H&E). (*B*) Areas of increased cellularity and occasional mitoses (H&E). GFAP (*C*) and OLIG2 (*D*) immunostains were diffusely positive and the tumor was negative for synaptophysin (*E*; highlights indicate entrapped axons and neurons). (*F*) A BCOR immunostain is positive in tumor nuclei.

RRAS2 mutations. All tumors lacked alterations in *IDH1*, *IDH2*, *H3F3A*, and *HIST1H3B/C*, as well as *TERT* and *PTEN*, and had low somatic mutation burden. Chromosomal copy number analysis of the high-grade gliomas in this cohort showed multiple chromosomal gains and losses per tumor, and their number was significantly higher than in spontaneous high-grade gliomas, suggesting that the copy number changes might happen somatically at the time of radiation.

PRACTICAL APPROACH TO THE DIAGNOSIS OF PEDIATRIC GLIOMAS

In a time when targeted therapy is available for a subset of pediatric gliomas and treatment options are evolving rapidly, the molecular features of a tumor are a pivotal component of a pathology report. Surgical specimens of gliomas are often limited and tissue triaging is the first important step in reaching a detailed but specific diagnosis. Tissue conservation and test selection are important. Ordering unstained slides upfront with no waste, separating a fragment of tissue into 2 blocks even if it can be accommodated in 1, avoiding immunostains that do not bring the case closer to a specific diagnosis (eg, GFAP in a clearly glial neoplasm, IDH1 in an infant) are just a few of the techniques that can be used to conserve material. Molecular test selection depends on tumor type: many pediatric gliomas harbor fusions between genes on the same chromosome, meaning that either a comprehensive fusion panel or a gene-specific fluorescence in situ hybridization probe, such as *BRAF*, *FGFR*, the *TRK* family of genes, *MYB*, *ALK1*, or *ROS1*, will be needed. Some targeted exome sequencing panels contain algorithms that investigate for the presence of fusions in a selected number of genes.[35] Although immunosurrogate markers for molecular alterations are useful in reaching a diagnosis, most clinical trial enrollments and targeted therapies require molecular confirmation of immunohistochemical findings.

Given the limited standard therapeutic options, particularly in high-grade gliomas and infantile gliomas, an integrated pathologic diagnosis that includes the histologic and molecular findings is of utmost importance in guiding clinical management.

REFERENCES

1. Curtin SC, Minino AM, Anderson RN. Declines in cancer rate deaths among children and adolescents in the United States, 1999-2014. NCHS Data Brief 2016;(257):1–8.
2. Ostrom QT, Gittleman H, Truitt G, et al. CBTRUS statistical report: primary brain and other central nervous system tumors diagnosed in the United States in 2011-2015. Neuro Oncol 2018; 20(suppl_4):iv1–86.
3. Louis DN, Ohgaki H, Wiestler OD, et al. WHO classification of tumours of the central nervous system. revised 4th edition. Geneva (Switzerland): WHO Press; 2016.
4. Ryall S, Tabori U, Hawkins C. A comprehensive review of paediatric low-grade diffuse glioma: pathology, molecular genetics and treatment. Brain Tumor Pathol 2017;34:51–61.
5. Jones DTW, Kieran MW, Alexandrescu S, et al. Pediatric low-grade gliomas: next biologically driven steps. Neuro Oncol 2018;20(2):160–73.
6. Bar EE, Lin A, Tihan T, et al. Frequent gains at chromosome 7q34 involving BRAF in pilocytic astrocytoma. J Neuropathol Exp Neurol 2008;67(9): 878–87.

7. Jones DT, Hutter B, Jager N, et al. Recurrent somatic alterations of FGFR1 and NTRK2 in pilocytic astrocytoma. Nat Genet 2013;45(8):927–32.
8. Pfister S, Janzarik WG, Remke M, et al. BRAF gene duplication constitutes a mechanism of MAPK pathway activation in low-grade astrocytomas. J Clin Invest 2008;118(5):1739–49.
9. Helgager J, Lidov HG, Mahadevan NR, et al. A novel GIT2-BRAF fusion in pilocytic astrocytoma. Diagn Pathol 2017;12(1):82.
10. Klintworth GK, garner A, editors. Garner and Klintworth's Pathobiology of ocular disease. 3rd edition. Boca Raton (FL): CRC Press; 2008.
11. Aoki Y, Niihori T, Narumi Y, et al. The RAS/MAPK syndromes: novel roles of the RAS pathway in human genetic disorders. Hum Mutat 2008;29(8):992–1006.
12. Burckhard C, Di Patre PL, Schuler D, et al. A population-based study of the incidence and survival rates in patients with pilocytic astrocytoma. J Neurosurg 2003;98(6):1170–4.
13. Stokland T, Liu JF, Ironside JW, et al. A multivariate analysis of factors determining tumor progression in childhood low-grade glioma: a population-based cohort study (CCLG CNS9702). Neuro Oncol 2010; 12(12):1257–68.
14. Collins VP, Jones DT, Giannini C. Pilocytic astrocytoma: pathology, molecular mechanisms and markers. Acta Neuropathol 2015;129(6):775–88.
15. Dias-Santagata D, Lam Q, Vernovsky K, et al. BRAF V600E mutations are common in pleomorphic xanthoastrocytoma: diagnostic and therapeutic implications. PLoS One 2011;6(3):e17948.
16. Weber RG, Hoischen A, Ehrler M, et al. Frequent loss of chromosome 9, homozygous CDKN2A/p14(ARF)/CDKN2B deletion and low TSC1 mRNA expression in pleomorphic xanthoastrocytomas. Oncogene 2007;26(7):1088–97.
17. Phillips JJ, Gong H, Chen K, et al. The genetic landscape of anaplastic pleomorphic xanthoastrocytoma. Brain Pathol 2019;29(1):85–96.
18. Phillips JJ, Gong H, Joseph NM, et al. Activating NRF1-BRAF and ATG7-RAF1 fusions in anaplastic pleomorphic xanthoastrocytoma without BRAF p.V600E mutation. Acta Neuropathol 2016;132(5): 757–60.
19. Alexandrescu S, Korshunov A, Lai SH, et al. Epithelioid glioblastomas and anaplastic epithelioid pleomorphic xanthoastrocytomas – same entity or first cousins? Brain Pathol 2016;26(2):215–23.
20. Korshunov A, Chavez L, Sharma T, et al. Epithelioid glioblastomas stratify into established diagnostic subsets upon integrated molecular analysis. Brain Pathol 2018;28(5):656–62.
21. Wang M, Tihan T, Rojiani AM, et al. Monomorphous angiocentric glioma: a distinctive epileptogenic neoplasm with features of infiltrating astrocytoma

and ependymoma. J Neuropathol Exp Neurol 2005; 64(1D):875–81.

22. Bandopadhayay P, Ramkissoon LA, Jain P, et al. MYB-QKI rearrangements in angiocentric glioma drive tumorigenicity through a tripartite mechanism. Nat Genet 2016;48(3):273–82.

23. D' Aronco L, Rouleau C, Gayden T, et al. Brainstem angiocentric gliomas with MYB-QKI rearrangements. Acta Neuropathol 2017;134(4):667–9.

24. Weaver KJ, Crawford LM, Bennett JA, et al. Brainstem angiocentric glioma: report of 2 cases. J Neurosurg Pediatr 2017;20(4):347–51.

25. Chan E, Bollen AW, Sirohi D, et al. Angiocentric glioma with MYB-QKI fusion located in the brainstem, rather than cerebral cortex. Acta Neuropathol 2017;134(4):671–3.

26. Lasorella A, Sanson M, Iavarone A. FGFR-TACC gene fusions in human glioma. Neuro Oncol 2017; 19(4):475–83.

27. Jones KA, Bossler AD, Bellizzi AM, et al. BCR-NTRK2 fusion in a low-grade glioma with distinctive morphology and unexpected aggressive behavior. Cold Spring Harb Mol Case Stud 2019;5(2), [pii: a003855].

28. Siegfried A, Rousseau A, Maurage CA, et al. EWSR1-PATZ1 gene fusion may define a new glioneuronal tumor entity. Brain Pathol 2019;29(1): 53–62.

29. Torre M, Meredith DM, Dubuc A, et al. Recurrent EP30-BCOR fusions in pediatric gliomas with distinct clinicopathologic features. J Neuropathol Exp Neurol 2019;78(4):305–14.

30. Huse JT, Snuderl M, Jones DT, et al. Polymorphous low-grade neuroepithelial tumor of the young (PLNTY): an epileptogenic neoplasm with oligodendroglioma-like components, aberrant CD34 expression, and genetic alterations involving the MAP kinase pathway. Acta Neuropathol 2017; 133(3):417–29.

31. Guerreiro Stucklin AS, Ryall S, Fukoka K, et al. Alterations in ALK/ROS1/NTRK/MET drive a group of infantile hemispheric gliomas. Nat Commun 2019; 10(1):4343.

32. Ferguson SD, Zhou S, Huse JT, et al. Targetable gene fusions associate with the IDH wild-type astrocytic lineage in adult gliomas. J Neuropathol Exp Neurol 2018;77(6):437–42.

33. Alvarez-Breckenridge C, Miller JJ, Nayyar N, et al. Clinical and radiographic response following targeting of BCAN-NTRK1 fusion in glioneuronal tumor. NPJ Precis Oncol 2017;1(1):5.

34. Johnson A, Severson E, Gay L, et al. Comprehensive genomic profiling of 282 pediatric low- and high-grade gliomas reveals genomic drivers, tumor mutational burden and hypermutation signatures. Oncologist 2017;22(12):1478–90.

35. Ramkissoon SH, Bandopadhayay P, Hwuang J, et al. Clinical targeted exome-based sequencing in combination with genome-wide copy number profiling: precision medicine analysis of 203 pediatric brain tumors. Neuro Oncol 2017;19(7):986–96.

36. Martinez-Lage M, Sahm F. Practical implications of the updated WHO classification of brain tumors. Semin Neurol 2018;38(1):11–8.

37. Zhang J, Wu G, Miller CP, et al. Whole-genome sequencing identifies genetic alterations in pediatric low-grade gliomas. Nat Genet 2013;45(6):602–12.

38. Ferris SP, Goode B, Joseph NM, et al. IDH1 mutation can be present in diffuse astrocytomas and giant cell glioblastomas of young children under 10 years of age. Acta Neuropathol. 2016;132(1): 153–5.

39. Brat DJ, Shehata BM, Casellano-Sanchez AA, et al. Congenital glioblastoma: a clinicopathologic and genetic analysis. Brain Pathol 2007;17(3): 276–81.

40. Junca A, Villalva C, Tachon G, et al. Crizotinib targets in glioblastoma stem cells. Cancer Med 2017; 6(11):2625–34.

41. Jones C, Karajannis MA, Joes DTW, et al. Pediatric high-grade glioma: biologically and clinically in need of new thinking. Neuro Oncol 2017;19(2): 153–61.

42. Sturm D, Witt H, Hovestadt V, et al. Hotspot mutations in H3F3A and IDH1 define distinct epigenetic and biological subgroups of glioblastoma. Cancer Cell 2012;22(4):425–37.

43. Buczoicz P, Hoeman C, Rakopoulos P, et al. Genomic analysis of diffuse intrinsic pontine gliomas identifies three molecular subgroups and recurrent activating ACVR1 mutations. Nat Genet 2014;46(5): 451–6.

44. Lewis PW, Muller MM, Koletsky MS, et al. Inhibition of PRC2 activity by a gain-of-function H3 mutation found in pediatric glioblastoma. Science 2013; 340(6134):857–61.

45. Castel D, Phillippe C, Calmon R, et al. Histone H3F3A and HIST1H3B K27M mutations define to subgroups of diffuse intrinsic pontine gliomas with different prognosis and phenotypes. Acta Neuropathol 2015;130(6):815–27.

46. Wu G, Broniscer A, McEachron TA, et al. Somatic histone H3 alterations in pediatric diffuse intrinsic pontine gliomas and non-brainstem glioblastomas. Nat Genet 2012;44(3):251–3.

47. Mackay A, Burford A, Carvalho D, et al. Integrated molecular meta-analysis of 1000 pediatric high-grade and diffuse intrinsic pontine glioma. Cancer Cell 2017;32(4):520–37.

48. Gessi M, Capper D, Sahm F, et al. Evidence of H3K27M mutations in posterior fossa ependymomas. Acta Neuropathol 2016;132(4):635–7.

49. Ryan S, Guzman M, Elbabaa SK, et al. H3K27M mutations are extremely rare in posterior fossa group A ependymoma. Childs Nerv Syst 2017;33(7): 1047–51.

50. Hochart A, Escande F, Rocourt N, et al. Long survival in a child with mutated K27M-H3.3 pilocytic astrocytoma. Ann Clin Transl Neurol 2015;2(4):439–43.

51. Orillac C, Thomas C, Dastagirzada Y, et al. Pilocytic astrocytoma and glioneuronal tumor with histone H3 K27M mutation. Acta Neuropathol Commun 2016; 4(1):84.

52. Pages M, Beccaria K, Boddaert N, et al. Co-occurrence of histone H3 K27M and BRAF V600E mutations in midline grade I ganglioglioma. Brain Pathol 2018;28(1):103–11.

53. Picca A, Berzero G, Bielle F, et al. FGFR1 actionable mutations, molecular specificities and outcome of adult midline gliomas. Neurology 2018;90(23): e2086–94.

54. Louis DN, Giannini C, Capper D, et al. cIMPACT-NOW update 2: diagnostic clarifications for diffuse midline glioma H3 K27M-mutant and diffuse astrocytoma/anaplastic astrocytoma, IDH-mutant. Acta Neuropathol 2018;135(4):639–42.

55. Jansen MH, Velduijzen van Zanten SE, Sanchez Aliaga E, et al. Survival prediction model of children with diffuse intrinsic pontine glioma based on clinical and radiological criteria. Neuro Oncol 2015;17(1): 160–6.

56. Hoffman LM, Veldhuijzen van Zanten SEM, Colditz N, et al. Clinical, radiologic, pathologic and molecular characteristics of long-term survivors of diffuse intrinsic pontine glioma (DIPG): a collaborative report from the International and European Society for Pediatric Oncology DIPG Registries. J Clin Oncol 2018;36(19):1963–72.

57. Bechet D, Gielen GG, Korshunov A, et al. Specific detection of methionine 27 mutation in histone 3 variants (H3K27M) in fixed tissue from high-grade astrocytomas. Acta Neuropathol 2014;128(5):733–41.

58. Bayliss J, Mukherjee P, Lu C, et al. Lowered H3K27me3 and DNA hypomethylation define poorly prognostic pediatric posterior fossa ependymomas. Sci Transl Med 2016;8(366):366ra161.

59. Mistry M, Zhukova N, Merico D, et al. BRAF mutation and CDKN2A deletion define a clinically distinct subgroup of childhood secondary high-grade glioma. J Clin Oncol 2015;33(9):1015–22.

60. Sturm D, Orr BA, Toprak UH, et al. New brain tumor entities emerge from molecular classification of CNS-PNETs. Cell 2016;164(5):1060–72.

61. Lopez GY, Van Ziffle J, Onodera C, et al. The genetic landscape of gliomas arising after therapeutic radiation. Acta Neuropathol 2019;137(1):139–50.

Embryonal Tumors of the Central Nervous System
An Update

Melissa M. Blessing, DO*, Sanda Alexandrescu, MD

KEYWORDS

- CNS embryonal tumors • Medulloblastoma • Embryonal tumor with multilayered rosettes
- Atypical teratoid rhabdoid tumor • High-grade neuroepithelial tumor

---

Key points

- Embryonal tumors of the Central Nervous System are a group of genetically heterogeneous WHO grade IV neoplasms.

- The understanding of their molecular biology is rapidly evolving and informs diagnosis, prognosis, and treatment options.

- Integration of the histology and molecular test results is essential for prognostic stratification and precise treatment of embryonal tumors.

- Careful tissue allocation for diagnostic and prognostic testing is essential.

- Embryonal tumors can signal the presence of germline tumor predisposition syndromes; interdisciplinary coordination is needed for assessment.

ABSTRACT

Embryonal tumors of the central nervous system (CNS) are rare, high-grade neoplasms predominantly affecting the pediatric population. Well-defined embryonal tumors include medulloblastoma, atypical teratoid/rhabdoid tumor, embryonal tumor with multilayered rosettes, C19MC-altered and embryonal tumor with multilayered rosettes, not otherwise specified, pineoblastoma, pituitary blastoma, CNS neuroblastoma, and ganglioneuroblastoma. Although their prognosis is nearly uniformly poor, the rapidly evolving understanding of their molecular biology contributes to diagnosis, prognosis, treatment, and clinical trial participation. Knowledge of current tumor stratification and diagnostic techniques will help pathologists guide care and preserve tissue for necessary or desired additional testing.

OVERVIEW

Central nervous system (CNS) embryonal tumors (ETs) include medulloblastoma, atypical teratoid rhabdoid tumor (AT/RT), embryonal tumor with multilayered rosettes (ETMR), pineoblastoma, pituitary blastoma, CNS neuroblastoma, ganglioneuroblastoma, and others, including embryonal tumors, not otherwise specified (NOS). They constitute fewer than 1% of all CNS neoplasms, and are seen most frequently between the ages of 0 to 4 years; they are slightly male-predominant.[1]

CNS ET can occur anywhere in the neuraxis. On MRI studies, they are contrast-enhancing, heterogeneous lesions with restricted diffusion due to their high cellularity. They can have necrotic foci, and may contain cysts. Although

---

Department of Pathology, Boston Children's Hospital, Harvard Medical School, 300 Longwood Avenue, Boston, MA 02115, USA
* Corresponding author.
E-mail address: Melissa.Blessing@Childrens.Harvard.Edu
Twitter: @DrMMB (M.M.B.)

Surgical Pathology 13 (2020) 235–247
https://doi.org/10.1016/j.path.2020.01.003
1875-9181/20/© 2020 Elsevier Inc. All rights reserved.

desmoplastic nodular medulloblastomas have a distinct radiographic appearance, most ETs have overlapping radiological features.[2,3] Many demonstrate leptomeningeal involvement and/or neuroaxis dissemination at the time of diagnosis.

The 2016 World Health Organization (WHO) classification of CNS tumors recommends a diagnosis that integrates the diagnostic (and often prognostic) molecular features when possible.[4] Appropriate molecular testing and standardized reporting are essential for prognosis and treatment, and also for clinical trial qualification and epidemiology.

MEDULLOBLASTOMA

Medulloblastomas (MBs) are posterior fossa ETs that constitute 20% of all childhood brain tumors,[1] and approximately 1% of primary CNS neoplasms in adults.[5,6] Imaging studies demonstrate a cerebellar vermis and/or brainstem, or cerebellar hemispheric mass that may involve the fourth ventricle and have leptomeningeal dissemination (Table 1).

MBs are classified into 4 histologic and 4 molecular groups. Histologically, MBs are subgrouped into classic, desmoplastic nodular, extensive nodularity, and anaplastic large cell morphology. All are diffusely positive for synaptophysin and can display scattered glial fibrillary acidic protein (GFAP)-positive cells. The Ki67 proliferation index is typically high, and INI1 immunopositivity excludes AT/RT. Representative illustrations of MB histology are depicted in Fig. 1.

Classic MB is characterized histologically by dense, small round blue cells with abundant mitoses and apoptosis. They may have Homer Wright rosettes, neurocytic differentiation, vague nodular areas, and other patterns. Classic MB is the largest histologic category and is seen in all molecular subgroups.

Desmoplastic nodular MBs have a characteristic appearance consisting of nodules of maturing neuroblasts in a background of abundant neuropil surrounded by a reticulin-rich network of mitotically active embryonal cells. Notably, this leads to a reversed pattern of staining with strong synaptophysin and low Ki67 in the neuropil-rich islands, and the reverse pattern in the surrounding primitive cells. Internodular-predominant GAB1 (cytoplasmic) and YAP1 (cytoplasmic and nuclear) positivity is typical.[7] Most desmoplastic nodular medulloblastomas have Sonic Hedgehog signaling pathway activation.

Medulloblastoma with extensive nodularity (MBEN) is characterized by an exaggerated desmoplastic nodular pattern with diminished intervening areas occupied by primitive neuroblasts. Their immunohistochemical and molecular profile mirrors desmoplastic nodular MBs.

Large cell/anaplastic medulloblastoma is a histologic subgroup characterized by frequent cells with marked atypia, cell-to-cell wrapping, cells 3 times larger than the surrounding ones, and atypical mitoses. Necrosis and confluent areas of apoptotic figures are frequent. This histologic type can have c*MYC* amplification, which, independently, is an indicator of poor prognosis. c*MYC*-amplified MBs present with leptomeningeal spread and/or distant metastasis in approximately 40% of cases.[8]

Two less common histologic variants include medulloblastoma with myogenic differentiation and medulloblastoma with melanocytic differentiation. These 2 variants do not carry independent prognostic implications. However, both *WNT* activation and *MYC* amplification have been reported in MBs with these morphologies.[9,10]

MOLECULAR SUBGROUPS

In 2012, an international consensus paper on expression profiling of medulloblastomas showed 4 discrete molecular subgroups with prognostic implications. These include Wnt pathway, Shh pathway, Group 3, and Group 4 medulloblastoma.[11] For practical clinical and prognostic purposes, the 2016 WHO classification of CNS tumors recommends the use of the histologic classification combined with the molecular classification. Because of differences in available modalities and sometimes the necessity for expression or methylation studies to accurately classify molecular groups 3 and 4, the WHO recommends the use of Wnt, Shh with and without *TP53* mutation, and non-Wnt/Shh molecular groups.[4,12,13]

WNT-activated (MB$_{WNT}$) MBs are the least common (10%) and are seen in older children and adults, and rarely in infants.[4] This molecular subgroup originates from the lower rhombic lip and dorsal brainstem, thus tumors are found along the foramen of Luschka attached to the cerebellar midline or brainstem and extending to the cerebellopontine angle, cisterna magna, or fourth ventricle.[3,14] MB$_{WNT}$ typically has classical morphology. Although beta-catenin is the widest available method to investigate for Wnt pathway activation, its interpretation can be sometimes difficult, as the extent of nuclear translocation varies from diffuse to less than 2% nuclei. Molecular confirmation of *CTNNB1* mutation, typically in exon 3, is recommended. Also, up to 85% of Wnt pathway–activated MBs have monosomy 6,

Table 1
Embryonal tumors of the central nervous system: imaging, histology, and molecular findings

Diagnosis	Location and Imaging Features	Key Histology and Immunohistochemistry	Molecular Alterations and Predisposition Syndromes
MB$_{WNT}$	Cerebellar midline, along Foramen of Luschka attached to the cerebellum or brainstem; may involve CP angle, cisterna magna, fourth ventricle	Classic histology, no significant LCA Positive: Neuroepithelial markers, INI1 (retained), Beta-catenin (nuclear & cytoplasmic), YAP1 (nuclear & cytoplasmic) Negative: GAB1, H3K27 M	Monosomy 6 *CTNNB1, DDX3X, TP53,* CSNK2B, *KMT2D, PIK3CA,EPHA7,* SWI/SNF subunits *(SMARCA4,ARID1A* and *ARID2)* In absence of *CTNNB1, APC* or *AXIN1* mutation (Germline or somatic) Turcot syndrome
MB$_{SHH}$	Cerebellar hemispheres; sometimes vermis DN/MBEN histology has "grapelike" imaging characteristics *TP53* mutant often have leptomeningeal spread	Wide histologic variety DN/MBEN histology is exclusive to MB$_{SHH}$ *TP53* mutant: Commonly LCA Positive: Neuroepithelial markers, INI1 (retained), YAP1 (nuclear and cytoplasmic) and GAB1 (cytoplasmic) Negative: Beta-catenin (cytoplasmic only), H3K27 M DN/MBEN: Internodular reticulin and high KI67; nodular strong synaptophysin and low KI67.	*TP53* wild-type MB$_{SHH}$: Chromosome 9q or 10q loss *PTCH1* or *SUFU* (germline or somatic), *SMO, GLI2 DDX3X, KMT2D; MYCN, MYCL* amplification Gorlin Syndrome *TP53* mutant MB$_{SHH}$: Chromosome 17p loss, chromothripsis TP53 point mutations (germline or somatic) GLI, MYCN, SHH amplification Li Fraumeni syndrome HAT complexes, *YAP1, BCOR,* rare *IDH1*R132 C, rare germline BRCA2 or PALB2 mutations Adults: PI3K/AKT/mTOR pathway, *TERT* promoter
MB$_3$	Cerebellar vermis near fourth ventricle	LCA or classic histology Positive: Neuroepithelial markers, INI1 (retained) Negative: Beta-catenin (cytoplasmic only), H3K27 M, YAP1, GAB1	Isodicentric chromosome 17 *MYC; MYC* or *MYCN* amplification *GFI1* or *GFI1B* alterations, *OTX2, KDM* family, *SMARC4, KBTBD4, CTDNEP1* and *KMT2D* Notch and TGFβ pathway alterations
MB$_4$	Cerebellar vermis	Positive: Neuroepithelial markers, INI1 (retained) Negative: Beta-catenin (cytoplasmic only), H3K27 M, YAP1, GAB1	Isodicentric chromosome 17 *MYCN* amplification *SNCAIP* duplication *GFI1* or *GFI1B* alterations, *KDM6A, SNCAIP, CDK6, ZMYM3* or *OTX2* Chromatin modification

Abbreviations: CP, cerebellopontine; DN, desmoplastic nodular; HAT, histone acetyltransferase; LoF, loss of function; MB$_3$, medulloblastoma group 3; MB$_4$, medulloblastoma group 4; MBEN, medulloblastoma with extensive nodularity; MB$_{SHH}$, Shh-activated medulloblastoma; MB$_{WNT}$, Wnt-activated medulloblastoma.

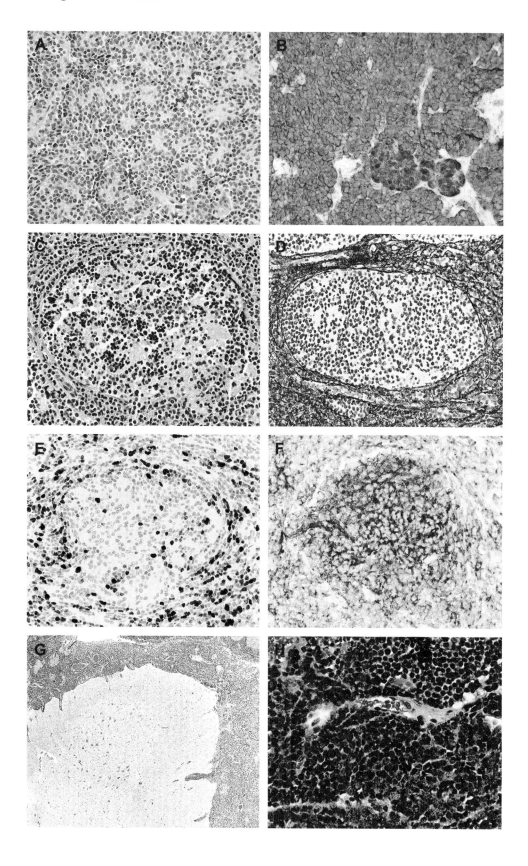

which is not seen in any of the other molecular subgroups. Secondary activation of the Sonic Hedgehog pathway has also been recently described; however, the prognostic significance of such findings is not clear.[15] Other co-occurring genetic events may include mutations in DDX3X, SMARCA4, KMT2D, TP53, KMT2D, PIK3CA, and EPHA7.[4,7,11] In up to 10% to 15% of cases, APC mutations activate the Wnt pathway instead of CTNNB1; evaluation for Turcot syndrome via germline analysis is indicated in these cases.[16,17]

WNT-activated medulloblastomas with classic morphology have an excellent prognosis in children. They have the lowest probability of metastatic disease, rarely recur, and have a 5-year survival rate of greater than 90%.[7,18] Rarely, large cell/anaplastic (LCA) features are observed; these have an uncertain prognosis.[4,7]

MB, SHH-activated (MB_SHH) constitutes approximately 30% of all MBs. MB_SHH is thought to originate from cerebellar granule neuron precursors, and involve the cerebellar hemispheres or vermis.[14] They are defined by Sonic Hedgehog pathway activation and further delineated by the presence or absence of TP53 mutation, which is prognostic in this subgroup. Histone acetyltransferase (HAT), YAP1, TERT, PRKAR1A, and IDH1R132 C alterations are also reported.[16,19] MB_SHH has the largest variety of morphology. Desmoplastic/nodular medulloblastoma and MBEN variants are most commonly associated with the MB_SHH subgroup; both have distinctive histologic and imaging features.[3]

MB_SHH wild-type TP53 has a bimodal age distribution, with most cases occurring in infants and young adults, and an equal sex distribution.[4] MBEN histology is exclusive to this group, and is seen in infants. Germline or somatic PTCH1 or SUFU mutations, or less commonly SMO or GLI2 alterations, activate the SHH pathway. Loss of chromosomes 9q or 10q, DDX3X or KMT2D mutation, MYCN or MYCL amplification, CSNK2B, EPHA7, and SWI/SNF subunit alterations may also be seen.[4,7,16,20] Individuals with Gorlin syndrome, particularly those with SUFU mutations, have a high risk of developing MB at a young age.[17,21]

TP53-wild-type tumors with desmoplastic nodular or MBEN histology are low-risk tumors, particularly in infants; classic morphology is standard risk, and LCAs have uncertain prognosis.[4]

MB_SHH with TP53 mutation is rare, and affects older children and teenagers.[22] In addition to TP53 mutations, MB_SHH can have GLI, MYC, MYCN, or SHH amplification, 17p loss, and chromothripsis.[4,23] Germline TP53 mutation testing, diagnostic of Li Fraumeni syndrome, should be considered.[4]

MB_SHH with TP53 mutation has worse prognosis, as it is unresponsive to therapy.[23] Those with classic and LCA histology are high-risk. Although less frequent than in MB_SHH TP53 wild-type, desmoplastic nodular histology is the most common histology in this subgroup and has an uncertain prognosis.[4]

MB group 3 (MB_3) constitutes approximately 20% of all MBs, but almost half of all cases in infants; they frequently (up to 45%) present with metastatic disease and affect boys more than girls.[11] This group is rare in adults.[20] Their origin is in neural stem cells, and they typically involve the cerebellar vermis near the fourth ventricle.[11,24] A subset of MB_3 has cMYC amplification, which portents an unfavorable outcome.[7,16,25] MB_3 has LCA or classic morphology and expresses the same neural markers as other MBs. They are negative for GAB1, YAP1, and nuclear beta-catenin.[7] Additional molecular alterations involve OTX2, KDM family, SMARC4, KBTBD4, CTDNEP1, and KMT2D.[16]

MB_3 has the worst prognosis of all MB groups, because of their high rate of metastatic disease and cMYC amplification.

MB group 4 (MB_4) is the largest group, constituting at least 40% of all MBs. They are most common in children and teenagers, and are 3 times more common in boys.[4] They are thought to arise from unipolar brush cells (upper rhombic lip), and are found in the cerebellar vermis.[14,24] MB_4 often exhibits classic morphology, but anaplasia may also be seen. In addition to isodicentric chromosome 17 and GFI1 or GFI1B alterations, MB_4 may have MYCN amplification and mutations involving KDM6A, SNCAIP, CDK6, ZMYM3, or OTX2.[16] In addition, 80% of the girls with MB_4 have loss of a

Fig. 1. Classic MB with small, round blue cells, Homer Wright rosettes, and numerous mitotic figures (A; 200x); MB_WNT demonstrate nuclear beta-catenin positivity, which may be very focal (B; 400x). Desmoplastic nodular MB with maturing neuroblasts and neuropil surrounded by embryonal cells (C; 400x) and desmoplasia (D; 400x). The nodules demonstrate low Ki67 (E; 400x) and strong synaptophysin positivity (F; 400x), while the surrounding less-differentiated component has the reverse pattern. MB often present with leptomeningeal spread and extend into parenchyma via perivascular (Virchow-Robin) spaces, as pictured in this cervical spinal cord section (G; 20x). LCA features may be patchy, and include notably larger neoplastic cells (bottom) which may also have prominent nuclei and/or cell-wrapping (H; 600x).

chromosome X, an alteration that is not encountered in any of the other molecular groups.

The prognosis of MB_4 is favorable with classic morphology, and uncertain in LCA morphology. Like MB_3, some present with metastatic disease. The significance of metastatic disease is less clear in MB_4 but is thought to be the main prognostic factor.[11,13]

Additional proposed MB molecular groups are based on DNA methylation profile studies of large pediatric cohorts. A European cohort performed molecular analysis of more than 400 childhood MBs and grouped them into prognostically significant categories by DNA methylation microarray. MB_{WNT} remained unchanged, MB_{SHH} was separated into infant and childhood categories, and the MB_3 and MB_4 groups were each split into low-risk and high-risk groups.[26]

A large international collaboration evaluated DNA methylation and gene expression together via similarity network fusion of more than 700 MBs and discovered 12 prognostically significant categories. Briefly, MB_{WNT} was split between children with monosomy 6 who had good prognosis, and adults with chromosome 6 diploidy and a worse prognosis. MB_{SHH} consisted of 4 groups divided roughly by age and in which *MYCN* amplification and *TP53* are key prognostic factors; among these, some adults were found to harbor *TERT* promoter mutations and have worse prognosis. MB_3 consisted of 3 groups roughly divided by age; one group had a higher frequency of *GFI1* and *GRI1B* oncogenes, and another was high-risk independent of *MYC* amplification. MB_4 consisted of 3 groups again split by age; groups had *MYCN* or *CDK6* amplification, or *SNCAIP* duplications.[19]

Analyses of non-WNT/non-SHH MBs is ongoing. One recent study combined data of the 3 preceding groups with their own, resulting in 8 distinct subtypes with prognostic significance within Groups 3 and 4, based on methylation profiles.[27] Current research is further elucidating MB biology and behavior using single-cell transcriptome analysis.[28,29] Given the fact that use of methylation is not widely spread in clinical settings and given the available treatment protocols for MB, the current practical approach is to separate MBs based on histology and 4 molecular groups, with an emphasis on investigating *cMYC* amplification and anaplastic histology.

ATYPICAL TERATOID/RHABDOID TUMOR

AT/RTs are rare WHO Grade IV tumors typically encountered in children younger than 2 years old, and constitute approximately 15% of ETs in children ≤14 years old.[1] AT/RTs have slight supratentorial predominance but can arise anywhere in the neuraxis, including in the pineal and pituitary glands regions, where they have been described in adults.[30–32] Approximately 25% of AT/RTs present with leptomeningeal involvement.[33,34] Histologically, they can be highly variable. Classically they are composed of sheets of cells with reniform or round eccentric nuclei, prominent nucleoli, and eosinophilic cytoplasm; necrosis, mitoses, and hemorrhage are common. However, they may have epithelial and/or mesenchymal differentiation, or be composed of small round blue cells without readily identifiable rhabdoid features. AT/RTs characteristically express focally immunomarkers of all cell lineages (smooth muscle actin, GFAP, synaptophysin, epithelial membrane antigen), and have loss of INI1, or, very rarely, loss of BRG1 immunoexpression.

At a molecular level, AT/RTs usually have homozygous deletion of *SMARCB1* (encoding for INI1 protein); less frequently, AT/RTs can have a combination of *SMARCB1* loss-of-function mutations and heterozygous deletion, or, very rarely, 2 loss-of-function mutations of *SMARCB1*.[35] Very rare cases with homozygous deletion or biallelic loss-of-function mutations involving *SMARCA4* (encoding the BRG1 protein) have been described.[36] Approximately 30% of individuals with rhabdoid tumors, including AT/RT, have rhabdoid tumor predisposition syndrome (RTPS).[21,35,37] This syndrome is characterized by germline alterations in the SWI/SNF chromatin remodeling complex involving *SMARCB1* (RTPS type 1) or *SMARCA4* (RTPS type 2), predisposing individuals to the development of multiple rhabdoid tumors at a young age following a second somatic alteration.[37] Germline testing is recommended in all patients with AT/RT, as carriers of *SMARCB*1 or *SMARCA4* mutation are at risk of developing rhabdoid tumors in other parts of the body as well.[21] Neurovascular hamartoma has been described as a cutaneous stigmata of rhabdoid tumor predisposition syndrome: Perez-Atayde and colleagues[38] reported 2 cases of infants who presented with congenital polypoid skin lesions. At microscopic examination, these skin lesions were characterized by a dermal proliferation of oval cells that expressed S100 and had loss of INI1, admixed with a disorganized network of vascular channels. These cutaneous lesions did not grow, and their histology appeared to be benign. At further imaging, the children were found to have rhabdoid tumors elsewhere in the body. In a recent case in practice, diagnosis of such a lesion led to incidental discovery of AT/RT and

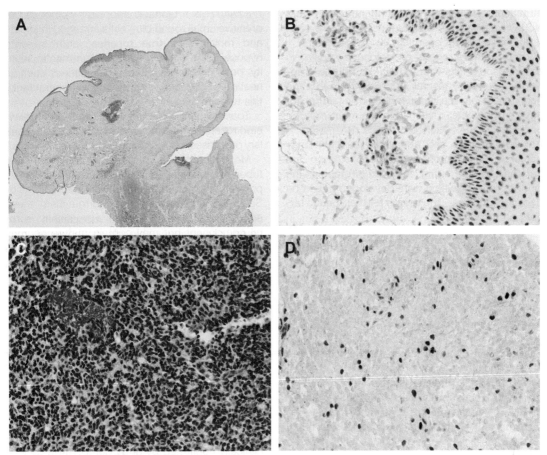

Fig. 2. Neurovascular hamartoma (*A*; 20x) with immunohistochemical loss of INI1 protein (*B*; 400x). ATRT in the same patient, composed of sheets of high grade neoplastic cells including scattered rhabdoid cells (*C*; 400x), and with immunohistochemical INI1 loss (*D*; 400x).

subsequent renal rhabdoid tumor in an infant (**Fig. 2**).

Additional AT/RT groups were proposed following a recent genetic and epigenetic study of pediatric AT/RTs that demonstrated 3 distinct molecular subgroups, summarized in **Table 2**.[39,40] The "ATRT-TYR" group is predominantly infratentorial; these AT/RTs are found in infants, and highly express TYR and other melanosomal markers. The "ATRT-MYC" group is mostly supratentorial, seen in older children, and overexpresses MYC and other HOX proteins. The methylation profile of adult sellar AT/RTs also cluster with this group.[31] The third proposed group, "ATRT-SHH," is seen approximately equally in both compartments, and is defined by

Table 2
Atypical teratoid rhabdoid tumor subgroups

Subgroups	Location	Methylation	Upregulated Pathways, Enhancers, and Enriched Transcription Factors
ATRT-TYR Melanogenesis	Infratentorial >> supratentorial	Hypermethylated	*TYR* or *DCT, MITF, CCND1, VEGFA, ERBB2,* ciliogenesis genes, *OTX2, LMX1A*
ATRT-MYC	Infratentorial > supratentorial	Hypomethylated	*MYC, REST,* HOX cluster genes, *ERBB2*
ATRT-SHH SHH pathway	Supratentorial = Infratentorial	Hypermethylated	*MYCN, GLI2, PTCH2, CDK6, FOXK1, ASCL1, HESS5/6, DLL 1/3*

mutations of genes impacting the Shh and NOTCH pathways. The prognosis of these subgroups has not yet been fully elucidated.

There are rare reports of prolonged survival in children and adults with AT/RT,[41,42] but the prognosis is generally dismal. In children, young age and metastasis are independent risk factors for adverse outcome; multimodal treatment may be beneficial in the absence of those risk factors.[41] Adjuvant therapy and additional resection may confer a better prognosis in adults, who are currently treated using standard protocols, the large majority of which were developed based on pediatric studies.[32] The search for therapeutic targets is ongoing.[43,44]

EMBRYONAL TUMOR WITH MULTILAYERED ROSETTES, C19MC-ALTERED AND EMBRYONAL TUMOR WITH MULTILAYERED ROSETTES, NOT OTHERWISE SPECIFIED

The discovery of chromosome 19 microRNA cluster amplification or fusion with *TTYH1* gene in a subset of tumors previously called embryonal tumor with abundant neuropil and true rosettes (ETANTR), ependymoblastoma, and medulloepithelioma led to their clustering under the entity ETMR,[45–48] included as an entity in the revised 2016 WHO Classification of Tumors of the Central Nervous System. They are most common in children under the age of 2 years.[4] ETMRs are predominantly seen in the cerebral hemispheres, but can be found anywhere in the neuraxis. They can become very large, extending to involve an entire or both hemispheres, and may be calcified and/or have cystic areas. All have pseudostratified, mitotically active true rosettes with neuroblasts (**Fig. 3**A, B). Three distinct histologic patterns are described as follows.

ETANTR is a biphasic neoplasm composed of primitive small round blue cells arranged in sheets and multilayered true rosettes, admixed with hypocellular areas of neuropil. High mitotic activity, positivity for neural stem cell markers such as nestin, CD99, and synaptophysin, characterize this tumor.[4]

Ependymoblastomas have clusters of multilayered rosettes and embryonal cells, some with fibrillary processes, but lack neuropil and ganglion cells.[4]

Medulloepitheliomas resemble primitive neural tubes. They have tubular, trabecular, and even papillary morphology with distinct, periodic acid-Schiff–positive membranes surrounding these epithelial structures. They lack a prominent neuropil component but may contain mature neurons and astrocytes in addition to embryonal cells, and some display melanin or mesenchymal features.[4] Medulloepithelioma histology warrants a separate, morphologic diagnosis, as the relative paucity of C19MC-alteration in this group suggests a distinct molecular mechanism yet to be elucidated.[4,49]

Aside from the alterations involving C19 MC, these tumors have recurrent copy number alterations of which gain of chromosome 2 is the most frequent; 7q and 11q gains, and 6q loss are also reported. LIN28 A antibody (**Fig. 3**C) is a sensitive immunosurrogate for C19 MC alterations, albeit not specific. The C19 MC alteration can be clinically confirmed by array comparative genetic hybridization. A co-occurring gain of chromosome 2 in this context is also highly suggestive of an ETMR, C19MC-altered.

Recently, Uro-Coste and colleagues[50] (2019) described 2 infants with cerebellar tumors that histologically resembled ETMR and had diffuse LIN28 immunopositivity, but contained heterologous elements (skeletal muscle differentiation in one case and cartilage in the other); both tumors lacked chromosome 19 alteration. On

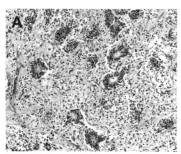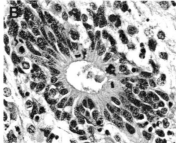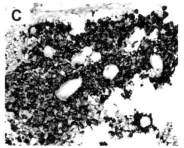

Fig. 3. ETMR, C19MC-altered with ETANTR morphology consisting of a (*A*; 100x) biphasic ET with prominent rosettes, which at higher power are distinguished by pseudostratified, multi-layered rosettes with basally oriented nuclei and numerous mitotic figures surrounding an empty (or amorphous fluid-filled) space (*B*; 400x). LIN28A immunostain is strong and diffusely positive (cytoplasmic) (*C*; 200x).

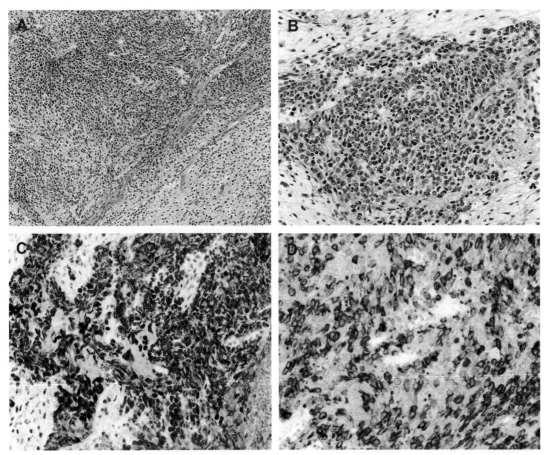

Fig. 4. ETMR-like ET with DICER1 mutation and lacking C19MC alteration composed of (*A*; 40x, *B*; 200x) prominent mutli-layered rosettes and demonstrating immunohistochemical retention of INI1 protein (*C*; 200x) and LIN28 immunopositivity (*D*; 200x).

methylome studies, these 2 tumors clustered separately from, but in close proximity to, ETMRs. Further molecular investigations showed biallelic mutations in the *DICER1* gene, 1 hotspot and 1 missense: a 2-hit mechanism identical to the ones seen in DICER1-associated tumors. An example of such a case is illustrated in **Fig. 4**.

The prognosis of ETMRs is dire. They recur, disseminate, and metastasize. The option of therapy targeting the mammalian target of rapamycin pathway was raised in a cell line study and supported in a subsequent mouse model.[51,52] The mainstay of treatment is still aggressive surgery and chemotherapy; even so, median survival is only a year.[52] Radiotherapy, particularly proton therapy, has recently been shown to prolong survival.[53]

PINEOBLASTOMA

Pineoblastomas (PBs) are poorly demarcated, frequently invasive pineal lesions occurring in the first 2 decades of life. They have typical ET morphology, variable Homer Wright and Flexner-Wintersteiner rosettes, and sometimes heterologous differentiation (**Fig. 5**A). CRX immunoreactivity (**Fig. 5**B), a marker of pineal or retinal origin, distinguishes these from other ETs of the CNS.[54]

The molecular background of PB is not fully elucidated. However, recent studies showed that genes involves in microRNA dysregulation, such as *DICER1* and *DROSHA* play an important role in their genesis, and are mutually exclusive.[55–57] PBs can be seen in the context of *DICER1* tumor predisposition syndrome, where the germline *DICER1* mutation is usually accompanied by loss of heterozygosity of the other allele. A smaller subset of DICER1-associated PBs has biallelic mutations in *DICER1*.[58] If available, DICER1 immunostain will show corresponding loss in the neoplastic cells of tumors with loss of heterozygosity. *DROSHA* is functionally upstream of *DICER1* in the microRNA pathway; homozygous *DROSHA* deletions are also described in PB.[56,58]

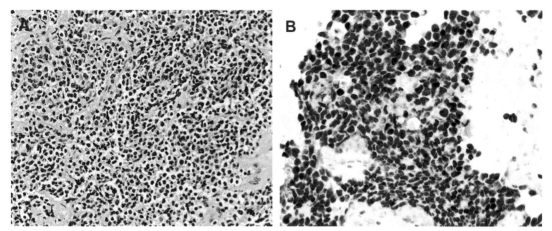

Fig. 5. Pineoblastoma with DICER1 mutation and (*A*; 200) typical ET morphology. CRX immunoreactivity is strong (*B*; 400), distinguishing it from metastatic pleuropulmonary blastoma; the latter is more common in the pediatric population.

In retinoblastoma syndrome, PB is a component of "trilateral retinoblastoma," along with bilateral retinoblastomas.[59]

Like other ETs, PB may present with disseminated disease (approximately 30%); their median survival ranges from 1 to 8 years.[4]

PITUITARY BLASTOMA

Pituitary blastoma is an exceedingly rare embryonal tumor occurring in infants and presenting with Cushing syndrome and diabetes insipidus. Histologically, it is composed of cells that resemble the blastic pituitary gland admixed with Rathke epithelial structures and folliculo-stellate cells.[60] Pituitary blastomas are immunopositive for ACTH and growth hormone, which is a rare combination in pituitary adenomas.

Pituitary blastomas have *DICER1* alterations (14 tested cases presented in literature) similar to those seen in PB, and are characteristic of DICER1 tumor predisposition syndrome.[57,58]

OTHER CENTRAL NERVOUS SYSTEM EMBRYONAL TUMORS

The shift away from histologic categorization and from the PNET bucket diagnostic term was prompted by several important studies showing distinct molecular alteration groupings.[49,61,62] The list of molecularly defined ETs continues to grow, informing diagnosis, prognosis, and treatment.[63–65]

A large international cohort generated DNA methylation profiles of more than 300 "CNS-PNETs" and compared them with a large reference sample. In addition to reclassifying numerous tumors, 4 new entities were discovered: CNS Ewing Sarcoma Family Tumor with *CIC* alteration, CNS High-Grade Neuroepithelial Tumor with *MN1* alteration, CNS High-Grade Neuroepithelial Tumor with *BCOR* alteration, and CNS Neuroblastoma with *FOXR2* (CNS NB-FOXR2) activation.[63] Of those, many have glial or uncertain origin, hence, for the purpose of this review, only CNS NB-FOXR2 activation is discussed.

CNS NB-FOXR2s are ETs morphologically similar to what is currently classified as CNS neuroblastoma (see the following). They have small cell morphology and express OLIG2 and synaptophysin; many contain neuropil and neurocytic or ganglion cells, Homer Wright rosettes, vascular pseudorosettes, and high mitotic activity. In addition to *FOXR2* alterations, chromosome 1q gain and 16q loss are seen.[63]

CNS neuroblastoma and *CNS ganglioneuroblastoma* are classified by the 2016 WHO as unique entities; both are WHO Grade IV. Both typically demonstrate necrosis with granular calcification and palisading and/or Homer Wright rosettes. CNS neuroblastoma exhibit neuropil and neurocytic cells that express neural markers, admixed with primitive cells, whereas CNS ganglioneuroblastomas have neurocytic cells and often-binucleate ganglion cells, and sheets of primitive cells.[4] The prognosis of these exceedingly rare tumors is not certain.

PRACTICE POINTS

At present time, CNS ETs are largely defined by their molecular alterations. Although immunosurrogates for protein products of mutations and other alterations are more widely used, most are not entirely specific. Therefore, molecular confirmation through DNA-based targeted exome sequencing, array comparative genomic hybridization (C19 MC amplification, for example) or fusion panels when needed, is necessary for a specific, reliable diagnosis that carries important prognostic and therapeutic implications. Methylation, a method of diagnostic clustering that gives copy number information, too, is popular in Europe, and some institutions in the United States have implemented it, albeit mostly as a research modality; it can be particularly helpful in the subclassification of CNS ETs.[16,19,26,27,31,39,40,46,56,63,66,67]

Aside from tissue utilization for a specific integrative diagnosis, almost each of these patients will eventually be enrolled in clinical trials and research protocols. Most pediatric brain tumor clinical trials require 20 to 30 unstained slides and frozen tissue, if available, for enrollment. Hence, mindfulness regarding tissue preservation is necessary, particularly if the specimens are small. Ways to preserve tissue include cutting unstained slides upfront to avoid facing the block multiple times, splitting tissue among multiple blocks to ensure that numerous sections can be cut, and avoiding immunostains that do not bring the case closer to a specific diagnosis meaningful to the patient's future treatment and prognosis. Knowledge of various molecular panels and if/how the result will impact diagnosis, prognosis, and/or treatment is equally important for conservation of tissue. Last, but possibly most important for patient care, seeking expert consultation and molecular testing at an outside institution (if not readily available) in a timely fashion can lead to more precise medical management and ability to participate in clinical trials.

DISCLOSURE

The authors have nothing to disclose.

REFERENCES

1. Ostrom QT, Gittleman H, Truitt G, et al. CBTRUS statistical report: primary brain and other central nervous system tumors diagnosed in the United States in 2011-2015. Neuro Oncol 2018; 20(suppl_4):iv1–86.
2. Shih RY, Koeller KK. Embryonal tumors of the central nervous system: from the radiologic pathology archives. Radiographics 2018;38(2):525–41.
3. Colafati GS, Voicu IP, Carducci C, et al. MRI features as a helpful tool to predict the molecular subgroups of medulloblastoma: state of the art. Ther Adv Neurol Disord 2018;11, 1756286418775375.
4. Louis DN, Ohgaki H, Wiestler OD. WHO classification of tumours of the central nervous system. Revised 4th edition. Lyon (France): International Agency for Research on Cancer (IARC); 2016.
5. Remke M, Hielscher T, Northcott PA, et al. Adult medulloblastoma comprises three major molecular variants. J Clin Oncol 2011;29(19):2717–23.
6. Zhao F, Ohgaki H, Xu L, et al. Molecular subgroups of adult medulloblastoma: a long-term single-institution study. Neuro Oncol 2016;18(7):982–90.
7. Ellison DW, Dalton J, Kocak M, et al. Medulloblastoma: clinicopathological correlates of SHH, WNT, and non-SHH/WNT molecular subgroups. Acta Neuropathol 2011;121(3):381–96.
8. Brown HG, Kepner JL, Perlman EJ, et al. "Large cell/anaplastic" medulloblastomas: a Pediatric Oncology Group Study. J Neuropathol Exp Neurol 2000; 59(10):857–65.
9. Rajeshwari M, Kakkar A, Nalwa A, et al. WNT-activated medulloblastoma with melanotic and myogenic differentiation: Report of a rare case. Neuropathology 2016;36(4):372–5.
10. Wright KD, von der Embse K, Coleman J, et al. Isochromosome 17q, MYC amplification and large cell/anaplastic phenotype in a case of medullomyoblastoma with extracranial metastases. Pediatr Blood Cancer 2012;59(3):561–4.
11. Taylor MD, Northcott PA, Korshunov A, et al. Molecular subgroups of medulloblastoma: the current consensus. Acta Neuropathol 2012;123(4): 465–72.
12. Jones DT, Jager N, Kool M, et al. Dissecting the genomic complexity underlying medulloblastoma. Nature 2012;488(7409):100–5.
13. Ramaswamy V, Remke M, Bouffet E, et al. Risk stratification of childhood medulloblastoma in the molecular era: the current consensus. Acta Neuropathol 2016;131(6):821–31.
14. Gibson P, Tong Y, Robinson G, et al. Subtypes of medulloblastoma have distinct developmental origins. Nature 2010;468(7327):1095–9.
15. Iorgulescu JB, Van Ziffle J, Stevers M, et al. Deep sequencing of WNT-activated medulloblastomas reveals secondary SHH pathway activation. Acta Neuropathol 2018;135(4):635–8.
16. Northcott PA, Buchhalter I, Morrissy AS, et al. The whole-genome landscape of medulloblastoma subtypes. Nature 2017;547(7663):311–7.
17. Waszak SM, Northcott PA, Buchhalter I, et al. Spectrum and prevalence of genetic predisposition in medulloblastoma: a retrospective genetic study and prospective validation in a clinical trial cohort. Lancet Oncol 2018;19(6):785–98.
18. Clifford SC, Lusher ME, Lindsey JC, et al. Wnt/Wingless pathway activation and chromosome 6 loss characterize a distinct molecular sub-group of

medulloblastomas associated with a favorable prognosis. Cell Cycle 2006;5(22):2666–70.

19. Cavalli FMG, Remke M, Rampasek L, et al. Intertumoral Heterogeneity within Medulloblastoma Subgroups. Cancer Cell 2017;31(6):737–54.e6.

20. Kool M, Korshunov A, Remke M, et al. Molecular subgroups of medulloblastoma: an international meta-analysis of transcriptome, genetic aberrations, and clinical data of WNT, SHH, Group 3, and Group 4 medulloblastomas. Acta Neuropathol 2012;123(4): 473–84.

21. Foulkes WD, Kamihara J, Evans DGR, et al. Cancer Surveillance in Gorlin Syndrome and Rhabdoid Tumor Predisposition Syndrome. Clin Cancer Res 2017;23(12):e62–7.

22. Kool M, Jones DT, Jager N, et al. Genome sequencing of SHH medulloblastoma predicts genotype-related response to smoothened inhibition. Cancer Cell 2014;25(3):393–405.

23. Zhukova N, Ramaswamy V, Remke M, et al. Subgroup-specific prognostic implications of TP53 mutation in medulloblastoma. J Clin Oncol 2013; 31(23):2927–35.

24. Vladoiu MC, El-Hamamy I, Donovan LK, et al. Childhood cerebellar tumours mirror conserved fetal transcriptional programs. Nature 2019;572(7767):67–73.

25. Lamont JM, McManamy CS, Pearson AD, Clifford SC, Ellison DW. Combined histopathological and molecular cytogenetic stratification of medulloblastoma patients. Clin Cancer Res 2004;10(16): 5482–93.

26. Schwalbe EC, Lindsey JC, Nakjang S, et al. Novel molecular subgroups for clinical classification and outcome prediction in childhood medulloblastoma: a cohort study. Lancet Oncol 2017;18(7):958–71.

27. Sharma T, Schwalbe EC, Williamson D, et al. Second-generation molecular subgrouping of medulloblastoma: an international meta-analysis of Group 3 and Group 4 subtypes. Acta Neuropathol 2019; 138(2):309–26.

28. Zhang L, He X, Liu X, et al. Single-cell transcriptomics in medulloblastoma reveals tumor-initiating progenitors and oncogenic cascades during tumorigenesis and relapse. Cancer Cell 2019; 36(3):302–18.e7.

29. Hovestadt V, Smith KS, Bihannic L, et al. Resolving medulloblastoma cellular architecture by single-cell genomics. Nature 2019;572(7767):74–9.

30. Paolini MA, Kipp BR, Sukov WR, et al. Sellar region atypical teratoid/rhabdoid tumors in adults: clinicopathological characterization of five cases and review of the literature. J Neuropathol Exp Neurol 2018;77(12):1115–21.

31. Johann PD, Bens S, Oyen F, et al. Sellar region atypical teratoid/rhabdoid tumors (ATRT) in adults display DNA methylation profiles of the ATRT-MYC subgroup. Am J Surg Pathol 2018;42(4):506–11.

32. Chan V, Marro A, Findlay JM, et al. A systematic review of atypical teratoid rhabdoid tumor in adults. Front Oncol 2018;8:567.

33. Hilden JM, Meerbaum S, Burger P, et al. Central nervous system atypical teratoid/rhabdoid tumor: results of therapy in children enrolled in a registry. J Clin Oncol 2004;22(14):2877–84.

34. Meyers SP, Khademian ZP, Biegel JA, et al, Zimmerman RA. Primary intracranial atypical teratoid/rhabdoid tumors of infancy and childhood: MRI features and patient outcomes. AJNR Am J Neuroradiol 2006;27(5):962–71.

35. Eaton KW, Tooke LS, Wainwright LM, et al. Spectrum of SMARCB1/INI1 mutations in familial and sporadic rhabdoid tumors. Pediatr Blood Cancer 2011;56(1): 7–15.

36. Hasselblatt M, Gesk S, Oyen F, et al. Nonsense mutation and inactivation of SMARCA4 (BRG1) in an atypical teratoid/rhabdoid tumor showing retained SMARCB1 (INI1) expression. Am J Surg Pathol 2011;35(6):933–5.

37. Sredni ST, Tomita T. Rhabdoid tumor predisposition syndrome. Pediatr Dev Pathol 2015;18(1):49–58.

38. Perez-Atayde AR, Newbury R, Fletcher JA, et al. Congenital "neurovascular hamartoma" of the skin. A possible marker of malignant rhabdoid tumor. Am J Surg Pathol 1994;18(10):1030–8.

39. Tegeder I, Thiel K, Erkek S, et al. Functional relevance of genes predicted to be affected by epigenetic alterations in atypical teratoid/rhabdoid tumors. J Neurooncol 2019;141(1):43–55.

40. Johann PD, Erkek S, Zapatka M, et al. Atypical teratoid/rhabdoid tumors are comprised of three epigenetic subgroups with distinct enhancer landscapes. Cancer Cell 2016;29(3):379–93.

41. von Hoff K, Hinkes B, Dannenmann-Stern E, et al. Frequency, risk-factors and survival of children with atypical teratoid rhabdoid tumors (AT/RT) of the CNS diagnosed between 1988 and 2004, and registered to the German HIT database. Pediatr Blood Cancer 2011;57(6):978–85.

42. Makuria AT, Rushing EJ, McGrail KM, et al. Atypical teratoid rhabdoid tumor (AT/RT) in adults: review of four cases. J Neurooncol 2008;88(3):321–30.

43. Phi JH, Sun CH, Lee SH, et al. NPM1 as a potential therapeutic target for atypical teratoid/rhabdoid tumors. BMC Cancer 2019;19(1):848.

44. Nesvick CL, Nageswara Rao AA, Raghunathan A, et al. Case-based review: atypical teratoid/rhabdoid tumor. Neurooncol Pract 2019;6(3):163–78.

45. Korshunov A, Remke M, Gessi M, et al. Focal genomic amplification at 19q13.42 comprises a powerful diagnostic marker for embryonal tumors with ependymoblastic rosettes. Acta Neuropathol 2010;120(2):253–60.

46. Korshunov A, Sturm D, Ryzhova M, et al. Embryonal tumor with abundant neuropil and true rosettes

(ETANTR), ependymoblastoma, and medulloepithelioma share molecular similarity and comprise a single clinicopathological entity. Acta Neuropathol 2014;128(2):279–89.

47. Nobusawa S, Yokoo H, Hirato J, et al. Analysis of chromosome 19q13.42 amplification in embryonal brain tumors with ependymoblastic multilayered rosettes. Brain Pathol 2012;22(5):689–97.

48. Li M, Lee KF, Lu Y, et al. Frequent amplification of a chr19q13.41 microRNA polycistron in aggressive primitive neuroectodermal brain tumors. Cancer Cell 2009;16(6):533–46.

49. Spence T, Sin-Chan P, Picard D, et al. CNS-PNETs with C19MC amplification and/or LIN28 expression comprise a distinct histogenetic diagnostic and therapeutic entity. Acta Neuropathol 2014;128(2):291–303.

50. Uro-Coste E, Masliah-Planchon J, Siegfried A, et al. ETMR-like infantile cerebellar embryonal tumors in the extended morphologic spectrum of DICER1-related tumors. Acta Neuropathol 2019;137(1):175–7.

51. Spence T, Perotti C, Sin-Chan P, et al. A novel C19MC amplified cell line links Lin28/let-7 to mTOR signaling in embryonal tumor with multilayered rosettes. Neuro Oncol 2014;16(1):62–71.

52. Schmidt C, Schubert NA, Brabetz S, et al. Preclinical drug screen reveals topotecan, actinomycin D, and volasertib as potential new therapeutic candidates for ETMR brain tumor patients. Neuro Oncol 2017;19(12):1607–17.

53. Jaramillo S, Grosshans DR, Philip N, et al. Radiation for ETMR: Literature review and case series of patients treated with proton therapy. Clin Transl Radiat Oncol 2019;15:31–7.

54. Santagata S, Maire CL, Idbaih A, et al. CRX is a diagnostic marker of retinal and pineal lineage tumors. PLoS One 2009;4(11):e7932.

55. Lee JC, Mazor T, Lao R, et al. Recurrent KBTBD4 small in-frame insertions and absence of DROSHA deletion or DICER1 mutation differentiate pineal parenchymal tumor of intermediate differentiation (PPTID) from pineoblastoma. Acta Neuropathol 2019;137(5):851–4.

56. Snuderl M, Kannan K, Pfaff E, et al. Recurrent homozygous deletion of DROSHA and microduplication of PDE4DIP in pineoblastoma. Nat Commun 2018;9(1):2868.

57. de Kock L, Sabbaghian N, Plourde F, et al. Pituitary blastoma: a pathognomonic feature of germ-line DICER1 mutations. Acta Neuropathol 2014;128(1):111–22.

58. de Kock L, Priest JR, Foulkes WD, et al. An update on the central nervous system manifestations of DICER1 syndrome. Acta Neuropathol 2019.

59. de Jong MC, Kors WA, de Graaf P, et al. Trilateral retinoblastoma: a systematic review and meta-analysis. Lancet Oncol 2014;15(10):1157–67.

60. Scheithauer BW, Horvath E, Abel TW, et al. Pituitary blastoma: a unique embryonal tumor. Pituitary 2012;15(3):365–73.

61. Schwalbe EC, Hayden JT, Rogers HA, et al. Histologically defined central nervous system primitive neuro-ectodermal tumours (CNS-PNETs) display heterogeneous DNA methylation profiles and show relationships to other paediatric brain tumour types. Acta Neuropathol 2013;126(6):943–6.

62. Picard D, Miller S, Hawkins CE, et al. Markers of survival and metastatic potential in childhood CNS primitive neuro-ectodermal brain tumours: an integrative genomic analysis. Lancet Oncol 2012;13(8):838–48.

63. Sturm D, Orr BA, Toprak UH, et al. New brain tumor entities emerge from molecular classification of CNS-PNETs. Cell 2016;164(5):1060–72.

64. Kram DE, Henderson JJ, Baig M, et al. Embryonal tumors of the central nervous system in children: the era of targeted therapeutics. Bioengineering (Basel) 2018;5(4).

65. Guerreiro Stucklin AS, Ramaswamy V, Daniels C, et al. Review of molecular classification and treatment implications of pediatric brain tumors. Curr Opin Pediatr 2018;30(1):3–9.

66. Capper D, Stichel D, Sahm F, et al. Practical implementation of DNA methylation and copy-number-based CNS tumor diagnostics: the Heidelberg experience. Acta Neuropathol 2018;136(2):181–210.

67. Halliday GC, Junckerstorff RC, Bentel JM, et al. The case for DNA methylation based molecular profiling to improve diagnostic accuracy for central nervous system embryonal tumors (not otherwise specified) in adults. J Clin Neurosci 2018;47:163–7.

Update on Circumscribed Gliomas and Glioneuronal Tumors

Jie Chen, MD, PhD[a], Sonika M. Dahiya, MBBS, MD[b],*

KEYWORDS

- Well-circumscribed • Glioma • Glioneuronal tumor • Benign • Low-grade

Key points

- Circumscribed intra-axial tumors are slow-growing and generally much more common in pediatric population as compared to their adult counterparts.
- Magnetic resonance imaging is critical for evaluation and particularly so in small biopsies.
- While molecular findings are distinct in some, *BRAF* alteration is common in the frequently occurring tumors and is shared across several histologic types.
- Neurofilament protein is a useful immunostain to illustrate the solid and infiltrative pattern, although a rapidly growing high-grade tumor can sometimes be expansile.
- Often contain dystrophic calcifications, perivascular chronic inflammatory infiltrate, Rosenthal material, and/or eosinophilic granular bodies. CD34 may be a good ancillary marker in glioneuronal processes.

ABSTRACT

Well-circumscribed intra-axial CNS tumors encompass a wide variety of gliomas and glioneuronal tumors, usually corresponding to WHO grades I and II. Nonetheless, sometimes high-grade 'diffuse' gliomas such as gliosarcoma and giant cell glioblastoma can be relatively circumscribed but are often found to have foci of diffuse infiltration on careful examination, harboring distinct molecular alterations. These tumors are excluded from the discussion in this chapter with the current review emphasizing on lower-grade entities to include a brief description of their histology and associated molecular findings. Like elsewhere in brain biopsy evaluation, imaging is crucial and acts as a surrogate to gross examination. Given the circumscribed nature of these tumors, surgery alone is the mainstay treatment in most entities.

CIRCUMSCRIBED ASTROCYTIC TUMORS

PILOCYTIC ASTROCYTOMA

Pilocytic astrocytoma is a well-circumscribed neoplasm (**Fig. 1**) frequently occurring in

[a] Department of Pathology and Microbiology, University of Nebraska Medical Center, 983135 Nebraska Medical Center, Omaha, NE 68198, USA; [b] Department of Pathology and Immunology, Washington University School of Medicine, 660 South Euclid Avenue, St Louis, MO 63110, USA
* Corresponding author.
E-mail address: sdahiya@wustl.edu

Surgical Pathology 13 (2020) 249–266
https://doi.org/10.1016/j.path.2020.02.004

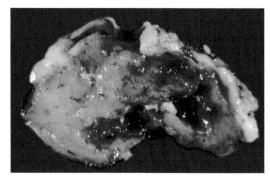

Fig. 1. Circumscribed glioma from a patient with pilocytic astrocytoma harboring predominantly solid and some cystic component.

children and young adults, with a predilection for the cerebellum. It also occurs in some other midline structures like the optic pathway ("optic pathway glioma," which is commonly associated with neurofibromatosis type I), hypothalamus, dorsal brain stem, spinal cord, and, rarely, cerebral hemispheres. Radiologically, classic pilocytic astrocytomas appear as a cystic mass with an enhancing mural nodule (**Fig. 2**A). Histologically, they often have a biphasic pattern with compact piloid areas intermixed with loose, microcystic areas. Rosenthal fibers and eosinophilic granular bodies are common (**Fig. 2**B). Mitotic activity is usually low. The blood vessels are often hyalinized with linear "glomeruloid" tufts of endothelial hyperplasia, sometimes making it challenging to differentiate from high-grade glioma. Glial fibrillary acidic protein (GFAP) is usually strongly and diffusely positive and highlights their long, hair-like (piloid) processes (**Fig. 3**). Molecularly, a majority of pilocytic astrocytomas are driven by alterations affecting the mitogen-activated protein kinase pathway. *BRAF–KIAA1549* fusion is the most common alteration in cerebellar pilocytic astrocytomas[1] and confers a better prognosis. These patients may also benefit from MEK/mammalian target of rapamycin (mTOR) inhibitor therapy.[2] Other fusions (*FAM131B–BRAF*,[3] *SRGAP3–RAF1*,[4] and *QK1–RAF1*[5]), mutations (*BRAFV600E*,[6] *KRAS*,[7] *FGFR1*, and *PTPN1*[8]), *NOTCH2* upregulation,[9] and *NF1* loss,[10] have also been reported infrequently. Pilocytic astrocytoma is a slow-growing, World Health Organization (WHO) grade I tumor with a 10-year overall survival rate of more than 95% after surgical resection alone.[11,12]

Key Features
PILOCYTIC ASTROCYTOMA

- Pilocytic astrocytoma can be sporadic or inherited; the inherited form is associated with neurofibromatosis 1
- Corresponds to WHO grade I
- Although the posterior fossa (PF) is the preferred site in patients with sporadic tumors, optic pathway gliomas are often seen in association with neurofibromatosis type I and tend to have infiltrative pattern
- Classic MRI appearance features a cyst with mural enhancing nodule
- Biphasic histology with compact areas enriched in piloid cells (rendering its name pilocytic), Rosenthal material, and loose microcystic areas with variable eosinophilic granular bodies
- Typically low proliferation indices although glomeruloid type microvascular proliferation is common and infarct-like necrosis may be seen
- Differential diagnoses include high-grade gliomas owing to microvascular proliferation and pleomorphism including multinucleate cells (pennies on a plate), glioneuronal tumors (like a complex dysembryoplastic neuroepithelial tumor [DNET] and ganglioglioma) owing to the predominance of glial component harboring a pilocytic phenotype
- *BRAF* fusion is much more frequent than *BRAF* point mutations

PILOMYXOID ASTROCYTOMA

Pilomyxoid astrocytoma is a variant of pilocytic astrocytoma that preferentially presents in the hypothalamus and optic chiasm in infants and young children (median age, 10 months). Histologically, it is characterized by an angiocentric arrangement of monomorphous, bipolar cells in a markedly myxoid background (**Fig. 4**). Pilomyxoid astrocytoma does not have Rosenthal fibers or eosinophilic granular bodies, and nuclear atypia is uncommon. Mitoses may be present, as is vascular proliferation. Necrosis is rare. The tumor cells demonstrate strong and diffuse reactivity for GFAP (**Fig. 5**) with perivascular accentuated staining, as well as stain for S100, and vimentin. BRAF V600E immunostain is usually negative. Pilomyxoid astrocytoma is genetically similar to pilocytic

A **B**

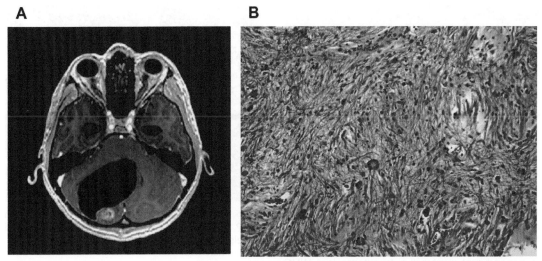

Fig. 2. Pilocytic astrocytoma. Cystic mass with mural enhancing nodule on T1-weighted postcontrast image (*A*). Predominance of compact areas in pilocytic astrocytoma with piloid and multinucleate cells (akin to pennies on a plate), rare microcyst with pale mucinous material, and abundant Rosenthal fibers in the background (*B*).

astrocytoma, and some of them show a *BRAF–KIAA1549* fusion.[13,14] Pilomyxoid astrocytomas are more aggressive than pilocytic astrocytomas with relatively frequent recurrences and cerebrospinal spread. However, it is unclear whether the aggressive behavior is related to its unfavorable hypothalamic/chiasmatic location. Therefore, the revised 2016 WHO classification[15] does not recommend a definitive grade for pilomyxoid astrocytoma.

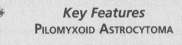

Key Features

PILOMYXOID ASTROCYTOMA

- Pilomyxoid astrocytoma is a variant of pilocytic astrocytoma, albeit with more frequent cerebrospinal fluid dissemination

- Typically presents in a suprasellar/hypothalamic location

- Angiocentric arrangement of relatively monomorphous tumor cells is characteristic, which can be further highlighted by GFAP stain

- Generally lacks Rosenthal material and eosinophilic granular bodies

SUBEPENDYMAL GIANT CELL ASTROCYTOMA

Subependymal giant cell astrocytoma is a slow-growing tumor that usually arises in the wall of

the lateral ventricles during the first 2 decades of life. It is seen in 5% to 15% of patients with confirmed tuberous sclerosis, a genetic disease caused by mutations in the *TSC1* or *TSC2* genes. The tumor is well-circumscribed, often calcified, contrast enhancing (**Fig. 6**A), and is composed of large ganglion-like to gemistocyte-like cells that are arranged in nests, fascicles, and sheets with dystrophic calcifications and mast cells in the background (**Fig. 6**B). Mitotic activity, endothelial proliferation, and necrosis are rare and are not indicative of anaplasia. The tumor cells show uniform immunoreactivity for S100, and variable immunoreactivity for GFAP and neuronal markers like synaptophysin and NeuN. CD34 is negative.

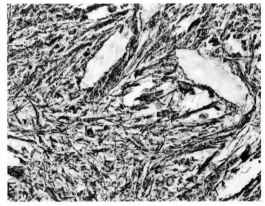

Fig. 3. Pilocytic astrocytoma. GFAP highlights long hairlike cytoplasmic processes.

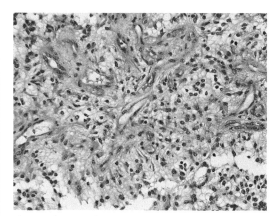

Fig. 4. Pilomyxoid astrocytoma. Angiocentric arrangement of tumor cells with myxoid matrix in the background.

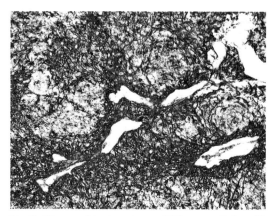

Fig. 5. Pilomyxoid astrocytoma. Diffuse reactivity with GFAP with accentuated staining around the blood vessels.

Subependymal giant cell astrocytoma is a WHO grade I tumor with a good prognosis when gross total resection is achieved.

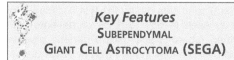

> ### *Key Features*
> #### Subependymal
> #### Giant Cell Astrocytoma (SEGA)
>
> - Mostly seen in association with tuberous sclerosis, where it can be the presenting feature
> - Can rarely be sporadic
> - Lateral ventricle most common site
> - Contrast enhancing on imaging
> - Variable expression of glial and neuronal markers
> - Often CD34 negative
> - Abundance of mast cells
> - Falls under the umbrella of "mTORopathy" owing to the activation of mTOR pathway
> - Corresponds to WHO grade I

PLEOMORPHIC XANTHOASTROCYTOMA AND ANAPLASTIC PLEOMORPHIC XANTHOASTROCYTOMA

Pleomorphic xanthoastrocytoma (PXA) is a rare epileptogenic astrocytic tumor that typically develops in the superficial cortical regions of children and young adults, most commonly in the temporal lobe. It is composed of large pleomorphic and frequently binucleated or multinucleated cells, spindled, and lipidized (xanthomatous) cells in a vaguely fascicular pattern (**Fig. 7**A). Eosinophilic granular bodies are almost always present

(**Fig. 7**B). A dense reticulin network is another histologic hallmark (**Fig. 8**A). By definition, mitotic activity is low (<5 mitoses per 10 high-power field), and necrosis is rare. GFAP is consistently expressed (**Fig. 8**B) and reactivity for neuronal markers may be negligible to patchy. A *BRAF* V600E mutation occurs in approximately 60% to 66% of PXA[6,16] and has potential therapeutic implications.[17] The combination of *BRAF V600E* mutation and absence of an *IDH* mutation favors the diagnosis of PXA over diffuse astrocytoma. A *CDKN2A/B* deletion is another frequent alteration in PXA that is not associated with tumor grade or *BRAF* mutation.[18,19] PXA is a WHO grade II tumor with a relatively favorable prognosis compared with diffuse astrocytoma (90.4% overall survival at 5 years[20]).

Anapalstic PXA is a PXA with 5 or more mitoses per 10 high-power fields and frequent necrosis; microvascular proliferation is relatively uncommon. Anaplasia may be focal in a tumor and manifest at first diagnosis or at time of recurrence. It is important to see conventional PXA areas before labeling a tumor as anaplastic PXA. The frequency of *BRAF V600E* mutation is lower among anaplastic PXA than among PXA. Anaplastic PXA is a WHO grade III tumor with a 5-year overall survival of 55.6%.[20]

> ### *Key Features*
> #### Pleomorphic Xanthoastrocytoma (PXA) and Anaplastic PXA
>
> - As the name implies, it is composed of highly pleomorphic and xanthic astrocytic cells
> - Usually supratentorial and associated with chronic seizure disorder

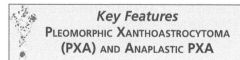

- Variable expression of glial and neuronal markers

- Variable fascicular arrangement of tumor cells with enrichment of reticulin fibers

- Perivascular chronic inflammatory cell infiltrate is common

- CD34 is a good ancillary marker, which shows variable staining from scattered to bushy to diffuse

- *BRAF* point mutations are seen in around two-thirds of tumors with a frequency that decreases to approximately 50% in anaplastic examples

- Corresponds to WHO grade II with anaplastic examples corresponding to WHO grade III

- Differential diagnoses includes high-grade tumors such as conventional glioblastoma, gliosarcoma, and epithelioid glioblastoma and can be rather challenging especially to distinguish from anaplastic PXA, particularly so when conventional PXA areas are not conspicuous

ANGIOCENTRIC GLIOMA

Angiocentric glioma is another low-grade, well-circumscribed, epileptogenic glioma of childhood and young adults. It is a cortically based tumor, most often involving supratentorial areas such as the temporal, frontal, or parietal lobes. Histologically, it consists of monomorphic, bland spindle cells oriented parallel or radial (ependymoma like) to blood vessels, with frequent subpial palisading.

Entrapped cortical neurons and neuropil can be present within the tumor, microscopically consistent with an infiltrative growth pattern. However, perineuronal satellitosis is rare, which is distinct from diffuse gliomas. The tumor cells are usually strongly positive for GFAP and S100. Some tumor cells show cytoplasmic dotlike reactivity for EMA and D2-40, resembling ependymoma. Recently, an *MYB-QKI* rearrangement was found to be a specific molecular alteration in angiocentric glioma.[21,22] Angiocentric glioma is a WHO grade I tumor and most cases can be cured by gross total resection with associated seizure control.

Key Features
ANGIOCENTRIC GLIOMA

- Epilepsy-associated tumor

- Often cortically based

- WHO grade I

- Monomorphic bipolar glial cells with perivascular pseudorosetted arrangement

- Expression of glial (GFAP: diffuse cytoplasmic) and ependymal markers (EMA and D2-40: perinuclear dotlike or ringlike pattern)

- Differential diagnoses includes ependymoma, diffuse glioma, and astroblastoma (especially when epithelioid cells are present, which is relatively rare)

- *MYB* rearrangement is frequent with *MYB:QKI* fusion being a common event

A

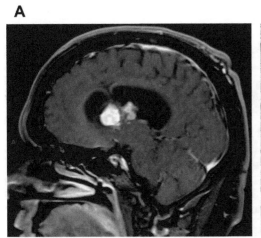

B

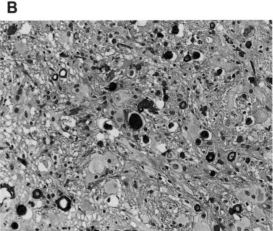

Fig. 6. Subependymal giant cell astrocytoma. A cystic mass with nodular areas of contrast enhancement arising from the ventricular wall of a patient with tuberous sclerosis (*A*). Numerous dystrophic calcifications, gemistocytic to ganglion-like cells, and spindled cells in subependymal giant cell astrocytoma (*B*).

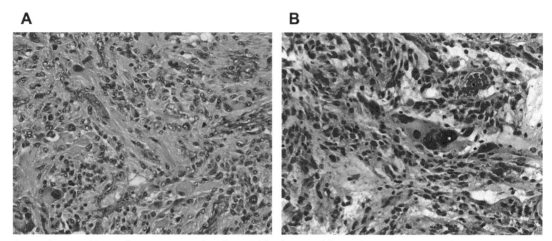

Fig. 7. Pleomorphic xanthoastrocytoma (PXA). Variable degree of fascicular arrangement of tumor cells is common in PXA (*A*). Large pleomorphic cells with several eosinophilic granular bodies in the background (*B*). Xanthic or lipidized cells may not always be present.

ASTROBLASTOMA

Astroblastoma is a rare, albeit another well-demarcated, glioma without clarity regarding its WHO grade at this time, typically seen in children and young adults, and often involving the supratentorial compartment.[23–26] It is generally characterized by glial cells with distinct cytoplasmic borders, arranged in conspicuous perivascular pseudorosetted to papillary architecture, harboring stouter cytoplasmic processes (**Fig. 9**A). Vascular hyalinization is frequent. Often positive, albeit variably, for GFAP (**Fig. 9**B) and lacks expression of epithelial markers. High-grade features constituted by dense cellularity, significant nuclear pleomorphism, increased mitotic activity, microvascular proliferation, and palisading necrosis have been reportedly associated with aggressive clinical behavior, although it has been questioned recently. Given the rarity of these tumors and challenges associated with accurate classification of these tumors, the molecular alterations are not as well-characterized; a relatively small series, however, has found frequent concomitant gains of chromosomes 19 and 20q.[27]

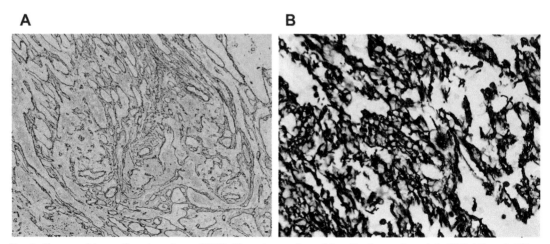

Fig. 8. Pleomorphic xanthoastrocytoma (PXA). There is usually a rich reticulin meshwork in PXA (*A*) and diffuse expression of GFAP (*B*).

Key Features
ASTROBLASTOMA

- Contrast-enhancing, supratentorial mass

- Usually seen in children and young adults

- Not yet assigned a specific WHO grade

- Pseudorosetted to papillary architecture, stouter glial processes, and hyalinized blood vessels

- Differential diagnoses includes ependymoma (delicate cytoplasmic processes, lack of hyalinized blood vessels as well as absence of epithelial marker expression, and the location aid distinguish it)

CHORDOID GLIOMA OF THE THIRD VENTRICLE

Chordoid glioma of the third ventricle is a well-circumscribed, solid, homogeneously contrast-enhancing tumor usually seen in third ventricle of adults. Benign-appearing epithelioid cells with abundant eosinophilic cytoplasm, discrete cytoplasmic borders, arranged in a chordoid arrangement with or without mucinous/myxoid stroma, robust lymphoplasmacytic cell infiltrate, and rare mitoses characterize it on histologic examination (**Fig. 10A**). These often demonstrate strong expression of GFAP (**Fig. 10B**) and CD34 with variable TTF1 reactivity[28] (**Fig. 10C**), which help its distinction from other chordoid tumors such as chordoma and chordoid meningioma. A recurrent point mutation in *PRKCA* (D463H) has recently

been identified as a consistent finding.[29] Long-term recurrence-free survival can be achieved through surgery alone, although the third ventricular location can make it challenging to attain a gross total resection.[30]

Key Features
CHORDOID GLIOMA
OF THE THIRD VENTRICLE

- Corresponds to WHO grade II

- Arises in the third ventricle of adults

- Epithelioid cells with or without myxoid/mucinous stroma, abundance of lymphoplasmacytic cell infiltrate, strong GFAP and TTF1 expression

- *PRKCA* (D463H) alteration is consistent

- Differential diagnoses include chordoma (physaliferous cells, bone involvement, brachyury reactivity, non-reactivity for TTF1 and GFAP) and chordoid meningioma (expresses EMA and PR, and lacks TTF1 and GFAP immunoreactivity)

POLYMORPHOUS LOW-GRADE NEUROEPITHELIAL TUMOR OF THE YOUNG

Polymorphous low-grade tumor of the young is a recently described tumor[31] in children and young adults with seizures, and is yet to make it to WHO classification scheme as a distinct

A

B

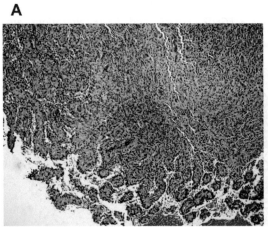

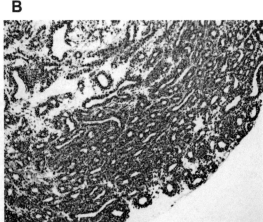

Fig. 9. Astroblastoma. Perivascular pseudorosetted to papillary arrangement of tumor cells with conspicuous hyalinized thickening of blood vessels (*A*) and strong reactivity for GFAP (*B*); the cytoplasmic processes are typically stouter.

A   B   C

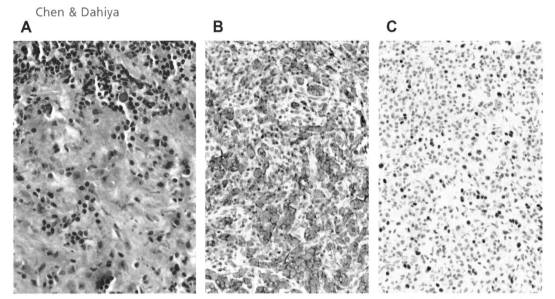

Fig. 10. Chordoid glioma of the third ventricle. Lack of fibrillar matrix and abundant lymphoplasmacytic infiltrate including few Russell bodies (*A*), strong GFAP (*B*) and variable TTF-1 (*C*) expression characterize chordoid glioma.

entity. It commonly presents in the superficial temporal lobe as a T2/fluid-attenuated inversion recovery hyperintense and calcified lesion without significant associated edema; infrequently enhances on postcontrast imaging. Its histology is characterized by relatively uniform appearing oligodendroglial cells with a diffuse growth pattern, thin capillary-sized vasculature and calcifications in the background, and an absence of concomitant dysmorphic neuronal component as well as Rosenthal material and eosinophilic granular bodies (**Fig. 11**A). CD34 (**Fig. 11**B) and OLIG2 (**Fig. 11**C) expression is usually strong and diffuse. GFAP expression is also common, albeit variable. Molecular alterations involving mitogen-activated protein kinase pathway ie, *FGFR2*, *FGFR3*, and *BRAF* genes are common.

> ### *Key Features*
> #### POLYMORPHOUS LOW-GRADE TUMOR OF THE YOUNG
>
> - Children and young adults
> - Commonly involves the temporal lobe
> - Epilepsy-associated tumor
> - Oligodendroglial cells in a diffuse growth pattern, lack of dysmorphic neurons, strong and diffuse expression of OLIG-2 and CD34
> - Not yet assigned a specific WHO entity and grade
> - Differential diagnoses include DNET (specific glioneuronal element), diffuse glioma (typically lacks diffuse CD34 immunoreactivity), ganglioglioma with predominance of oligodendroglioma component (presence of dysmorphic neuronal component)
> - *FGFR2*, *FGFR3*, and *BRAF* alterations are frequent

A   B   C

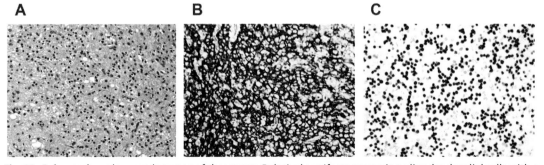

Fig. 11. Polymorphous low-grade tumor of the young. Relatively uniform appearing oligodendroglial cells with a diffuse growth pattern, lacking dysmorphic neuronal component and significant mitotic activity (*A*). Diffuse concomitant expression of CD34 (*B*) and OLIG-2 (*C*) is characteristic.

A   B   C

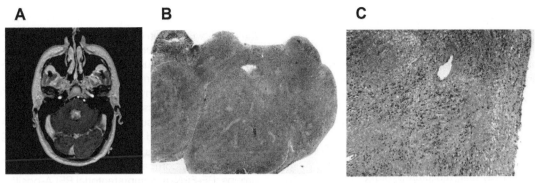

Fig. 12. Subependymoma. Slow-growing contrast-enhancing subependymoma of the fourth ventricle (*A*). Usually, these tumors are incidentally detected. Vaguely nodular architecture with acellular and paucicellular zonation highlighted on low power (*B*). Note the lack of true or pseudorosettes and hyalinization of the blood vessels (*C*). This tumor can sometimes have a microvascular proliferation.

EPENDYMAL TUMORS

SUBEPENDYMOMA

Subependymoma is a slow-growing, exophytic, intraventricular neoplasm that most frequently is found incidentally in the fourth ventricle in middle-aged and elderly patients, contrast enhancement is uncommon (**Fig. 12**A). Histologically, subependymoma is lobulated and well-demarcated, and is characterized by clusters of small, bland, uniform glial cells in a dense fibrillary matrix with frequent microcysts. Pseudorosettes and/or true rosettes are absent (**Fig. 12**B, C). Mitotic figures are rare and the blood vessels are often hyalinized. Because of their slow-growing nature, they are frequently associated with variable piloid gliosis in the surrounding tissue that is enriched in Rosenthal material and can be a diagnostic pitfall (**Fig. 13**). The tumor cells are usually immunoreactive for GFAP, and only rarely for EMA (in contrast to classic ependymoma). Subependymoma is a WHO grade I tumor with excellent prognosis after resection.[32]

> ### *Key Features*
> #### SUBEPENDYMOMA
>
> - Often incidental
> - Usually nonenhancing
> - Fourth ventricle
> - Middle aged and elderly
> - Acellular and hypocellular regions with uniform nuclei and hyalinized blood vessels
> - WHO grade I
> - Differential diagnoses may include a conventional ependymoma (presence of rosettes) and pilocytic astrocytoma (biphasic pattern with piloid cells)

MYXOPAPILLARY EPENDYMOMA

Myxopapillary ependymoma is an ependymal neoplasm that occurs almost exclusively in the conus medullaris, cauda equina, and filum terminale. The tumor cells have characteristically elongate fibrillary processes arranged in radial patterns around blood vessels (**Fig. 14**), which frequently demonstrate mucoid/myxoid degeneration, a feature that can be further highlighted by Alcian blue stain (**Fig. 15**). Immunoreactivity for GFAP is often diffuse. Reactivity for EMA, S100, CD99, and vimentin is also frequent. Based on a recent study on ependymomas across different anatomic sites using DNA methylation profiles, myxopapillary ependymoma is characterized by chromosomal instability with frequent DNA copy number alterations.[33] Myxopapillary ependymoma is a WHO grade I tumor with a 5-year overall survival rate of more than 95% after resection.[33–35]

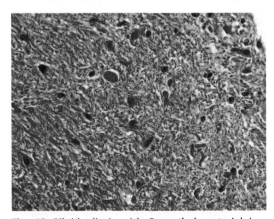

Fig. 13. Piloid gliosis with Rosenthal material is a frequent finding in the vicinity of a subependymoma owing to its slow-growing nature and can be a diagnostic pitfall.

Key Features
MYXOPAPILLARY EPENDYMOMA

- Commonly arise in cauda equina, and filum terminale of adults
- Frequently well-encapsulated
- Homogeneously contrast enhancing
- Perivascular mucoid/myxoid change, which can be highlighted by Alcian blue stain
- Corresponds to WHO grade I
- Anaplastic changes are extremely rare

EPENDYMOMA AND ANAPLASTIC EPENDYMOMA

Ependymoma is a circumscribed glioma in both children and adults that occurs mainly intracranially, and less frequently in the spinal cord. It is composed of small uniform cells with round nuclei and speckled chromatin in a fibrillary matrix. Pseudorosettes (tumor cells radially arranged around blood vessels forming perivascular anucleate zones) are frequent (**Fig. 16**A). Ependymal rosettes (tumor cells arranged around a central lumen) are another diagnostic feature, but these are less common. Perinuclear dot-like immunoreactivity for EMA (**Fig. 16**B) and D2-40 is typical in ependymomas. GFAP immunoreactivity is frequent in perivascular tumor cells, and may be variable in other areas of the tumor.

A histologically classic ependymoma is a WHO grade II tumor. When an ependymoma demonstrates high cellularity, elevated mitotic activity, widespread microvascular proliferation, and necrosis, it is considered an anaplastic ependymoma, which corresponds to a WHO grade III

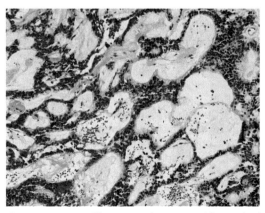

Fig. 14. Myxopapillary ependymoma with marked mucinous/myxoid change in the blood vessel walls.

tumor. However, clinical outcome of an ependymoma primarily depends not on histologic grade, but on the extent of surgical resection, adjuvant radiation therapy, and molecular group.

A recent DNA methylation profiling study of 500 ependymomas across 3 main central nervous system compartments, supratentorial brain (ST), posterior fossa (PF), and spine (SP), has identified 9 molecular subgroups of ependymomas, 3 from each anatomic compartment.[33] Among the 9 subgroups, PF-EPN-A or supratentorial RELA-positive ependymomas (discussed elsewhere in this article) show dismal prognosis. The PF-EPN-A subgroup accounting for about 74% of PF ependymomas, predominantly occur in the lateral PF in infants and young children (median age 3 years), and demonstrate a relatively balanced genome with widespread epigenomic alterations, including DNA CpG island hypermethylation, global DNA hypomethylation, and H3K27me3 loss with poor prognosis.[36–38] Much more recently, a subset of spinal ependymoma harboring *MYCN* amplification have been shown to be associated with poor prognosis.[39]

Key Features
EPENDYMOMA

- Posterior fossa (PF) common site
- PF-A is frequent in infants with H3 K27me3 loss and is associated with poor prognosis
- Supratentorial examples often have *RELA* fusion and are associated with a worse prognosis
- Perivascular pseudorosettes are characteristic with delicate cytoplasmic processes; true rosettes are "hallmark" but are infrequent
- Often GFAP positive and show perinuclear dot-like reactivity with EMA and D2-40
- Differential diagnoses includes oligodendroglioma (diffuse growth pattern, IDH mutant and 1p19q-codeleted) and central neurocytoma (lack of true or pseudorosettes and expression of neuronal markers) for the clear cell variant of ependymoma

EPENDYMOMA, *RELA* FUSION POSITIVE

Ependymoma, *RELA* fusion positive is a new entity in the 2016 updated WHO, and accounts for approximately 70% of childhood supratentorial tumors.[33] It does not have a specific morphology,

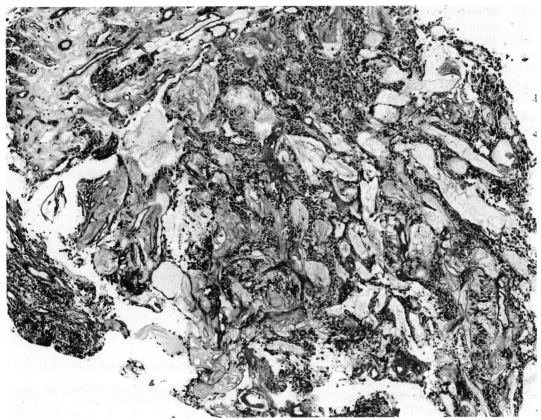

Fig. 15. Myxopapillary ependymoma. Alcian blue-PAS stain highlights the abundance of myxoid change within the vascular walls, partially rendering its name.

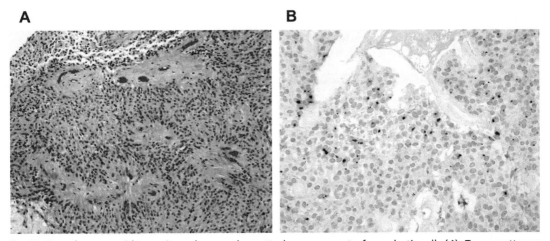

Fig. 16. Ependymoma with a perivascular pseudorosetted arrangement of neoplastic cells (*A*). True rosettes are rather infrequent but when present are diagnostic. Typically express both glial (GFAP; diffuse cytoplasmic) and epithelial markers (perinuclear dotlike). Shown is perinuclear dotlike intracytoplasmic reactivity for epithelial membrane antigen (*B*). D2-40 also shows a similar staining pattern to that of an EMA, but is generally slightly more widespread.

but is rather defined by the presence of *RELA* fusion, most commonly *C11orf95-RELA*, which can be detected by interphase fluorescence in situ hybridization with break-apart probes. *C11orf95-RELA* fusion is caused by a local chromosome shattering event (chromothripsis) on chromosome 11, and this fusion leads to constitutive activation of the nuclear factor-κB pathway. RELA-fused ependymoma is associated with different chromosomal copy number changes and molecular alterations compared to non–*RELA*-fused ependymomas.[40] *RELA* fusion-positive ependymomas have the worst prognosis of the 3 supratentorial molecular groups.

CIRCUMSCRIBED GLIONEURONAL TUMORS

DYSEMBRYOPLASTIC NEUROEPITHELIAL TUMOR

Dysembryoplastic neuroepithelial tumor (DNET) is a benign, predominantly cortically based glioneuronal neoplasm that most frequently occurs in the temporal lobe of children or young adults. Patients usually present with medically refractory focal epilepsy before the age of 20 years. The tumor presents as T2-hyperintense single or multiple pseudocysts on MRI, and typically has a multinodular character. Histologically, simple DNET shows a multinodular growth pattern with a specific glioneuronal element demonstrated by columns of axons oriented perpendicularly to the cortical surface. These columns are further surrounded by small uniform oligodendrocyte-like cells in a myxoid background, and bland-appearing neurons seem to float in the mucin-rich matrix (**Fig. 17**). In complex DNET, specific glioneuronal element is present together with glial nodules, which have histologic features of

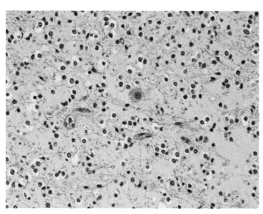

Fig. 17. DNET. Pools of pale mucin with uniform oligodendroglial cells and bland-appearing floating neurons.

pilocytic astrocytoma, ganglioglioma, diffuse glioma or other glial neoplasms. Dystrophic microcalcifications are common. Cortical dysplasia may be present in the surrounding brain parenchyma. The oligodendrocyte-like cells in DNET show immunoreactivity for OLIG-2, but not for GFAP or MAP2. DNET lacks an *IDH1/IDH2* mutation and 1p19q co-deletions. Instead, they often harbor germline or somatic *FGFR1* mutations.[41,42] These features help distinguish DNET from a diffuse glioma. DNET is a WHO grade I tumor with an excellent prognosis after surgery.

> ### Key Features
> ### DYSEMBRYOPLASTIC NEUROEPITHELIAL TUMOR (DNET)
>
> - Most common chronic seizure disorder
> - Corresponds to WHO grade I
> - Often cystic, multinodular, and cortically based tumor on imaging; can show contrast enhancement
> - Simple and complex forms
> - Pools of pale mucin with oligodendroglial-like cells and floating neurons
> - *FGFR1* alterations are frequent with lack of *IDH* mutation
> - Differential diagnoses includes oligodendroglioma (lacks "floating neurons"), ganglioglioma (absence of specific glioneuronal elements), and pilocytic astrocytoma (lacks neuronal elements)

GANGLIOGLIOMA AND ANAPLASTIC GANGLIOGLIOMA

Ganglioglioma is a slow-growing, most common epileptogenic glioneuronal tumor, predominantly occurring in the temporal lobe of children and young adults. They often present as intracortical cysts with a contrast-enhancing nodule on imaging, sometimes with associated calcifications. Ganglioglioma is a biphasic tumor with variable dysplastic neurons and neoplastic glial cells. Dysplastic neurons may be clumped or haphazardly arranged, and may show binucleation or multinucleation, cytomegaly, pale or vacuolated cytoplasm, abnormal distribution of Nissl substance, or disoriented processes. The glial component may resemble pilocytic astrocytoma, diffuse astrocytoma, or oligodendroglioma. Ganglioglioma frequently exhibits dense perivascular

A

B

C

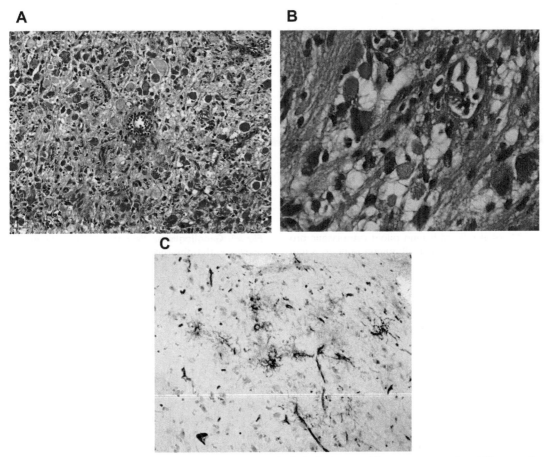

Fig. 18. Ganglioglioma. Dysmorphic ganglion cells and glial elements with numerous eosinophilic granular bodies and perivascular chronic inflammatory cell infiltrate (*A*). High power with better illustration of dysmorphic ganglion cells (*B*). CD34-positive spider cells characterized by highly ramified cytoplasmic processes are seen in the surrounding brain parenchyma with cortical dysplasia (*C*).

lymphocytic infiltrates and dystrophic calcification. Eosinophilic granular bodies are more often encountered than Rosenthal fibers (**Fig. 18**A, B). Patients with these tumors also have associated focal cortical dysplasia, which can be furthermore highlighted by CD34 (**Fig. 18**C) immunostain. The neoplastic glial cells are immunoreactive for GFAP (**Fig. 19**). Dysplastic neurons or ganglionic cells are immunoreactive for neurofilament (**Fig. 20**A), synaptophysin (**Fig. 20**B), chromogranin, and CD34 (**Fig. 21**). About 20% to 60% of gangliogliomas harbor a *BRAF* V600 E mutation.[6,43–45] The presence of this alteration in pediatric patients has been shown to be associated with a poor prognosis.[46] Gains of chromosomes 5, 6, and 7, and *CDKN2A* homozygous deletion have also been reported.[43,47] Ganglioglioma corresponds to WHO grade I with a good prognosis after surgical resection.

Key Features
GANGLIOGLIOMA

- Mesial temporal lobe is common site

- Mostly in children, and young adults with chronic seizure disorder

- Corresponds to WHO grade I

- Composed of glial and neuronal components with frequent perivascular chronic inflammatory cell infiltrate, and eosinophilic granular bodies

- *BRAF* point mutations are seen in around half of cases

- Differential diagnoses includes pilocytic astrocytoma (lack of dysmorphic neuronal component), diffuse glioma (contains entrapped native neurons highlighted by NeuN rather than dysmorphic/dysplastic neuronal elements that are highlighted by synaptophysin and neurofilament), and complex DNET (lacks substantial neuronal dysmorphism and chronic inflammatory cell infiltrate)

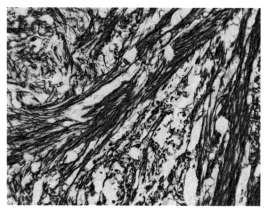

Fig. 19. Glial cells with long piloid cytoplasmic processes highlighted by a GFAP immunostain in a ganglioglioma with predominant pilocytic astrocytoma–like areas within the glial component.

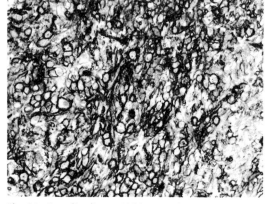

Fig. 21. Ganglioglioma. Widespread CD34 immunoreactivity within the tumor cells.

DESMOPLASTIC INFANTILE ASTROCYTOMA AND GANGLIOGLIOMA

Desmoplastic infantile astrocytoma (DIA) and desmoplastic infantile ganglioglioma (DIG) are rare neoplasms that occur in infants and young children (median age, 6 months). They often present as superficial, large, cystic lesions in the frontoparietal region. Histologically, DIA is composed of a prominent desmoplastic stroma admixed with spindled or gemistocytic astrocytes in a fascicular or storiform pattern. In DIG, besides the neoplastic astrocytes, there are also neoplastic neuronal cells with variable differentiation (**Fig. 22**A). Both DIA and DIG may have a poorly differentiated, small blue cell component (**Fig. 22**B). Although

dystrophic calcifications are often present, perivascular chronic inflammatory cell infiltrate is generally absent. In both DIA and DIG, there is a prominent reticulin-positive network in the desmoplastic stroma (**Fig. 22**C). The neoplastic astrocytes are immunoreactive for GFAP (**Fig. 22**D), the neuronal cells are positive for neuronal markers like synaptophysin (**Fig. 22**E), and the poorly differentiated neuroepithelial component reacts with both GFAP and neuronal markers. Mitotic activity and necrosis may be present in the poorly differentiated neuroepithelial component, but do not seem to influence prognosis. A recent study revealed somatic *BRAF* mutations in more than 40% of DIA/DIG,[48] most frequently *BRAF* V600E mutation. DIA and DIG are WHO grade I tumors with long-term survival after gross total resection.[49,50]

A   **B**

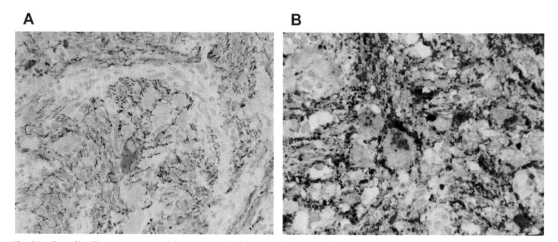

Fig. 20. Ganglioglioma. Dysmorphic neurons highlighted by neurofilament staining of their soma (*A*). Strong synaptophysin reactivity within dysplastic neurons (*B*).

Key Features
Desmoplastic Infantile Astrocytoma (DIA) and Desmoplastic Infantile Ganglioglioma (DIGG)

- Corresponds to WHO grade I
- Large, superficial, cerebral hemispheric, cystic masses in infants
- Composed of glial with or without neuronal elements in a robust desmoplastic background which can be highlighted by a reticulin stain
- *BRAF* point mutations are frequent
- Differential diagnoses includes PXA (presence of xanthic or lipidized cells, perivascular chronic inflammatory cell infiltrate and lack of small blue cells) and ganglioglioma (devoid of desmoplasia)

PAPILLARY GLIONEURONAL TUMOR

Papillary glioneuronal tumor (PGNT) is a rare, circumscribed, cystic or solid contrast-enhancing tumor that preferentially locates in the periventricular white matter of the temporal lobe in young adults. Histologically, it is characterized by pseudopapillary structures with hyalinized blood vessels, lined by flat to cuboidal astrocytes. Neurocytes and occasional ganglion cells are present in the interpapillary regions. The glial component is immunoreactive for GFAP or Olig2, and the neuronal component is positive for synaptophysin and NeuN. Recent studies have demonstrated that PGNT exhibits a characteristic methylation profile

and fusions involving *PRKCA*, most frequently an *SLC44S1-PRKCA* fusion.[51–53] PGNT is a WHO grade I tumor with a good prognosis.[54]

Key Features
Papillary Glioneuronal Tumor (PGNT)

- Corresponds to WHO grade I
- Generally presents as solid and cystic enhancing temporal lobe mass in young adults
- Pseudopapillary architecture with surrounding glial cells reactive for GFAP or OLIG-2 and presence of neuronal elements (neurocytic in nature) outside of glial cells which are seen immediately around the blood vessels
- Fusions involving *PRKCA* gene is a frequent molecular alteration
- Differential diagnoses includes extraventricular neurocytoma (lack of pseudopapillary architecture, much more uniform cells, paucity of glial processes, widespread expression of neuronal marker such as synaptophysin), astroblastoma (pseudorosetted architecture is rendered by perpendicular stouter cytoplasmic processes rather than parallel processes seen in PGNT as well as presence of hyalinized vasculature), ependymoma (absence of dysmorphic neuronal component) and rarely ganglioglioma (conspicuous dysmorphic ganglion cells and perivascular chronic inflammatory cell infiltrate, lack of pseudopapillary architecture, hyalinized vessels, and neurocytic elements)

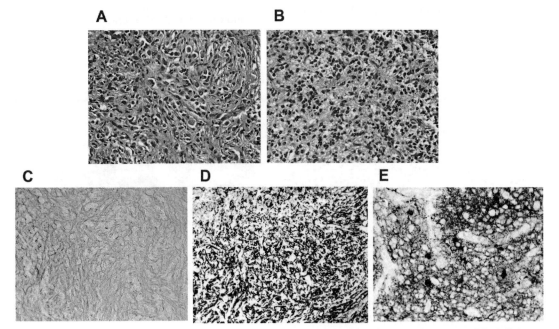

Fig. 22. DIG. Glial and dysmorphic neuronal elements are present in a fibrotic appearing stroma (*A*). Cellular appearing areas with high nuclear cytoplasmic ratio (somewhat blue cells) can be appreciated in some examples (*B*). Rich reticulin meshwork (*C*) with widespread expression of GFAP (*D*) and neuronal marker, synaptophysin (*E*).

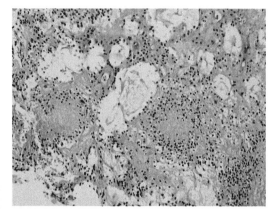

Fig. 23. RGNT with conspicuous rosetted architecture characterized by central neuropil which is surrounded by relatively uniform-appearing neurocytic cells. Also appreciated are microcysts that can characterize some cases.

such as GFAP. In contrast, the neurocytic cells immediately surrounding the central neuropil are generally strongly reactive for synaptophysin (**Fig. 24**B). They may also have oligodendroglioma-like or DNET-like areas. Although morphologically similar, RGNTs are distinct from pilocytic astrocytomas because they do not harbor *BRAF-KIAA1549* fusion or *BRAF V600E* mutation. Instead, a recent study has identified *FGFR1* mutation in 100%, *PIK3CA* mutation in 63%, and *NF1* mutation in 33% of RGNTs. This means RGNTs are characterized by combined genetic alterations affecting both mitogen-activated protein kinase and PI3K pathways.[56] RGNT is a WHO grade I tumor with a good prognosis.[55]

ROSETTE-FORMING GLIONEURONAL TUMOR

Rosette-forming glioneuronal tumor (RGNT) is a circumscribed, slow-growing tumor that typically arises in the fourth ventricle of young adults (median age, 22.5 years[55]). Histologically, it is a biphasic tumor with distinct neuronal and glial components. The neuronal component consists of small round bland neurocytes forming rosettes or perivascular pseudorosettes in a fibrillary background with or without microcysts (**Figs. 23** and **24A**). The glial component is usually composed of spindled cells that resemble those of pilocytic astrocytoma and can be highlighted by glial marker

Key Features
ROSETTE-FORMING GLIONEURONAL TUMOR (RGNT)

- Corresponds to WHO grade I

- Composed of glial and neuronal (neurocytic) components

- Fourth ventricle is preferred site but can occur in third ventricle

- Rosettes are formed by central neuropil with surrounding neurocytic cells

- *FGFR1* alterations are common

- Differential diagnoses includes pilocytic astrocytoma (lacks the neuropil-rich rosettes and often has *BRAF* alteration)

A

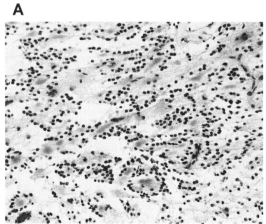

B

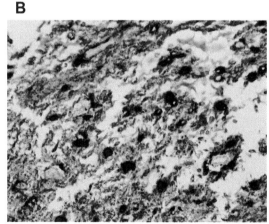

Fig. 24. RGNT. High-power showing neurocytic cells arranged in a rosetted arrangement (*A*). The central neuropil of rosettes is highlighted by its strong reactivity with synaptophysin (*B*).

DISCLOSURE

The authors have nothing to disclose.

REFERENCES

1. Jones DT, Kocialkowski S, Liu L, et al. Tandem duplication producing a novel oncogenic BRAF fusion gene defines the majority of pilocytic astrocytomas. Cancer Res 2008;68(21):8673–7.
2. Fangusaro J, Onar-Thomas A, Young Poussaint T, et al. Selumetinib in paediatric patients with BRAF-aberrant or neurofibromatosis type 1-associated recurrent, refractory, or progressive low-grade glioma: a multicentre, phase 2 trial. Lancet Oncol 2019;20(7):1011–22.
3. Cin H, Meyer C, Herr R, et al. Oncogenic FAM131B-BRAF fusion resulting from 7q34 deletion comprises an alternative mechanism of MAPK pathway activation in pilocytic astrocytoma. Acta Neuropathol 2011;121(6):763–74.
4. Jones DTW, Kocialkowski S, Liu L, et al. Oncogenic RAF1 rearrangement and a novel BRAF mutation as alternatives to KIAA1549:BRAF fusion in activating the MAPK pathway in pilocytic astrocytoma. Oncogene 2009;28(20):2119–23.
5. Zhang J, Wu G, Miller CP, et al. Whole-genome sequencing identifies genetic alterations in pediatric low-grade gliomas. Nat Genet 2013;45(6): 602–12.
6. Schindler G, Capper D, Meyer J, et al. Analysis of BRAF V600E mutation in 1,320 nervous system tumors reveals high mutation frequencies in pleomorphic xanthoastrocytoma, ganglioglioma and extracerebellar pilocytic astrocytoma. Acta Neuropathol 2011;121(3):397–405.
7. Collins VP, Jones DT, Giannini C. Pilocytic astrocytoma: pathology, molecular mechanisms and markers. Acta Neuropathol 2015;129(6):775–88.
8. Jones DT, Hutter B, Jager N, et al. Recurrent somatic alterations of FGFR1 and NTRK2 in pilocytic astrocytoma. Nat Genet 2013;45(8):927–32.
9. Tchoghandjian A, Fernandez C, Colin C, et al. Pilocytic astrocytoma of the optic pathway: a tumour deriving from radial glia cells with a specific gene signature. Brain 2009;132(Pt 6):1523–35.
10. Listernick R, Ferner RE, Liu GT, et al. Optic pathway gliomas in neurofibromatosis-1: controversies and recommendations. Ann Neurol 2007;61(3):189–98.
11. Burkhard C, Di Patre PL, Schuler D, et al. A population-based study of the incidence and survival rates in patients with pilocytic astrocytoma. J Neurosurg 2003;98(6):1170–4.
12. Mathew RK, O'Kane R, Parslow R, et al. Comparison of survival between the UK and US after surgery for most common pediatric CNS tumors. Neuro Oncol 2014;16(8):1137–45.
13. Lin A, Rodriguez FJ, Karajannis MA, et al. BRAF alterations in primary glial and glioneuronal neoplasms of the central nervous system with identification of 2 novel KIAA1549:BRAF fusion variants. J Neuropathol Exp Neurol 2012;71(1):66–72.
14. Colin C, Padovani L, Chappe C, et al. Outcome analysis of childhood pilocytic astrocytomas: a retrospective study of 148 cases at a single institution. Neuropathol Appl Neurobiol 2013;39(6):693–705.
15. Louis DN, Ohgaki H, Wiestler OD, et al. World Health Organization histological classification of tumours of the central nervous system. Lyon, France: International Agency for Research on Cancer; 2016.
16. Dias-Santagata D, Lam Q, Vernovsky K, et al. BRAF V600E mutations are common in pleomorphic xanthoastrocytoma: diagnostic and therapeutic implications. PLoS One 2011;6(3):e17948.
17. Hofer S, Berthod G, Riklin C, et al. BRAF V600E mutation: a treatable driver mutation in pleomorphic xanthoastrocytoma (PXA). Acta Oncol 2016;55(1): 122–3.
18. Weber RG, Hoischen A, Ehrler M, et al. Frequent loss of chromosome 9, homozygous CDKN2A/p14(ARF)/CDKN2B deletion and low TSC1 mRNA expression in pleomorphic xanthoastrocytomas. Oncogene 2007;26(7):1088–97.
19. Vaubel RA, Caron AA, Yamada S, et al. Recurrent copy number alterations in low-grade and anaplastic pleomorphic xanthoastrocytoma with and without BRAF V600E mutation. Brain Pathol 2018;28(2):172–82.
20. Ida CM, Rodriguez FJ, Burger PC, et al. Pleomorphic xanthoastrocytoma: natural history and long-term follow-up. Brain Pathol 2015;25(5):575–86.
21. Qaddoumi I, Orisme W, Wen J, et al. Genetic alterations in uncommon low-grade neuroepithelial tumors: BRAF, FGFR1, and MYB mutations occur at high frequency and align with morphology. Acta Neuropathol 2016;131(6):833–45.
22. D'Aronco L, Rouleau C, Gayden T, et al. Brainstem angiocentric gliomas with MYB-QKI rearrangements. Acta Neuropathol 2017;134(4):667–9.
23. Ahmed KA, Allen PK, Mahajan A, et al. Astroblastomas: a Surveillance, Epidemiology, and End Results (SEER)-based patterns of care analysis. World Neurosurg 2014;82(1–2):E291–7.
24. Bonnin JM, Rubinstein LJ. Astroblastomas: a pathological study of 23 tumors, with a postoperative follow-up in 13 patients. Neurosurgery 1989;25(1): 6–13.
25. Sughrue ME, Choi J, Rutkowski MJ, et al. Clinical features and post-surgical outcome of patients with astroblastoma. J Clin Neurosci 2011;18(6):750–4.
26. Merfeld EC, Dahiya S, Perkins SM. Patterns of care and treatment outcomes of patients with astroblastoma: a National Cancer Database analysis. CNS Oncol 2018;7(2):CNS13.

27. Brat DJ, Hirose Y, Cohen KJ, et al. Astroblastoma: clinicopathologic features and chromosomal abnormalities defined by comparative genomic hybridization. Brain Pathol 2000;10(3):342–52.

28. Bielle F, Villa C, Giry M, et al. Chordoid gliomas of the third ventricle share TTF-1 expression with organum vasculosum of the lamina terminalis. Am J Surg Pathol 2015;39(7):948–56.

29. Rosenberg S, Simeonova I, Bielle F, et al. A recurrent point mutation in PRKCA is a hallmark of chordoid gliomas. Nat Commun 2018;9(1):2371.

30. Desouza RM, Bodi I, Thomas N, et al. Chordoid glioma: ten years of a low-grade tumor with high morbidity. Skull Base 2010;20(2):125–38.

31. Huse JT, Snuderl M, Jones DT, et al. Polymorphous low-grade neuroepithelial tumor of the young (PLNTY): an epileptogenic neoplasm with oligodendroglioma-like components, aberrant CD34 expression, and genetic alterations involving the MAP kinase pathway. Acta Neuropathol 2017; 133(3):417–29.

32. Jain A, Amin AG, Jain P, et al. Subependymoma: clinical features and surgical outcomes. Neurol Res 2012;34(7):677–84.

33. Pajtler KW, Witt H, Sill M, et al. Molecular classification of ependymal tumors across all CNS compartments, histopathological grades, and age groups. Cancer Cell 2015;27(5):728–43.

34. Woehrer A, Hackl M, Waldhor T, et al. Relative survival of patients with non-malignant central nervous system tumours: a descriptive study by the Austrian Brain Tumour Registry. Br J Cancer 2014;110(2):286–96.

35. Lin Y, Smith ZA, Wong AP, et al. Predictors of survival in patients with spinal ependymoma. Neurol Res 2015;37(7):650–5.

36. Mack SC, Witt H, Piro RM, et al. Epigenomic alterations define lethal CIMP-positive ependymomas of infancy. Nature 2014;506(7489):445–50.

37. Bayliss J, Mukherjee P, Lu C, et al. Lowered H3K27me3 and DNA hypomethylation define poorly prognostic pediatric posterior fossa ependymomas. Sci Transl Med 2016;8(366):366ra161.

38. Panwalkar P, Clark J, Ramaswamy V, et al. Immunohistochemical analysis of H3K27me3 demonstrates global reduction in group-A childhood posterior fossa ependymoma and is a powerful predictor of outcome. Acta Neuropathol 2017;134(5):705–14.

39. Ghasemi DR, Sill M, Okonechikov K, et al. MYCN amplification drives an aggressive form of spinal ependymoma. Acta Neuropathol 2019;138(6):1075–89.

40. Torre M, Alexandrescu S, Dubuc AM, et al. Characterization of molecular signatures of supratentorial ependymomas. Mod Pathol 2020;33(1):47–56.

41. Rivera B, Gayden T, Carrot-Zhang J, et al. Germline and somatic FGFR1 abnormalities in dysembryoplastic neuroepithelial tumors. Acta Neuropathol 2016;131(6):847–63.

42. Trisolini E, Wardighi DE, Giry M, et al. Actionable FGFR1 and BRAF mutations in adult circumscribed gliomas. J Neurooncol 2019;145(2):241–5.

43. Pekmezci M, Villanueva-Meyer JE, Goode B, et al. The genetic landscape of ganglioglioma. Acta Neuropathol Commun 2018;6(1):47.

44. Chappe C, Padovani L, Scavarda D, et al. Dysembryoplastic neuroepithelial tumors share with pleomorphic xanthoastrocytomas and gangliogliomas BRAF(V600E) mutation and expression. Brain Pathol 2013;23(5):574–83.

45. Dougherty MJ, Santi M, Brose MS, et al. Activating mutations in BRAF characterize a spectrum of pediatric low-grade gliomas. Neuro Oncol 2010;12(7):621–30.

46. Dahiya S, Haydon DH, Alvarado D, et al. BRAF V600E mutation is a negative prognosticator in pediatric ganglioglioma. Acta Neuropathol 2013;125:901–10.

47. Prabowo AS, van Thuijl HF, Scheinin I, et al. Landscape of chromosomal copy number aberrations in gangliogliomas and dysembryoplastic neuroepithelial tumours. Neuropathol Appl Neurobiol 2015; 41(6):743–55.

48. Wang AC, Jones DTW, Abecassis IJ, et al. Desmoplastic Infantile Ganglioglioma/Astrocytoma (DIG/DIA) Are Distinct Entities with Frequent BRAFV600 Mutations. Mol Cancer Res 2018;16(10):1491–8.

49. Taratuto AL, Monges J, Lylyk P, et al. Superficial cerebral astrocytoma attached to dura. Report of six cases in infants. Cancer 1984;54(11):2505–12.

50. Cohen AR. The great neurosurgical masquerader: 3 cases of desmoplastic infantile ganglioglioma. J Neurosurg Pediatr 2019;1–9. https://doi.org/10.3171/2019.5.PEDS19151.

51. Hou Y, Pinheiro J, Sahm F, et al. Papillary glioneuronal tumor (PGNT) exhibits a characteristic methylation profile and fusions involving PRKCA. Acta Neuropathol 2019;137(5):837–46.

52. Nagaishi M, Nobusawa S, Matsumura N, et al. SLC44A1-PRKCA fusion in papillary and rosette-forming glioneuronal tumors. J Clin Neurosci 2016;23: 73–5.

53. Pages M, Lacroix L, Tauziede-Espariat A, et al. Papillary glioneuronal tumors: histological and molecular characteristics and diagnostic value of SLC44A1-PRKCA fusion. Acta Neuropathol Commun 2015;3:85.

54. Zhao RJ, Zhang XL, Chu SG, et al. Clinicopathologic and neuroradiologic studies of papillary glioneuronal tumors. Acta Neurochir (Wien) 2016;158(4):695–702.

55. Anyanwu CT, Robinson TM, Huang JH. Rosette-forming glioneuronal tumor: an update. Clin Transl Oncol 2019. https://doi.org/10.1007/s12094-019-02179-8.

56. Sievers P, Appay R, Schrimpf D, et al. Rosette-forming glioneuronal tumors share a distinct DNA methylation profile and mutations in FGFR1, with recurrent co-mutation of PIK3CA and NF1. Acta Neuropathol 2019;138(3):497–504.

Molecular Diagnostics in Lymphoid Neoplasms of the Central Nervous System

David M. Meredith, MD, PhD

KEYWORDS

• CNS lymphoma • Molecular diagnostics • Genomic • DLBCL

Key points

- Diffuse large B cell lymphoma (DLBCL) is the most common and most aggressive of the primary lymphoid neoplasms arising within the central nervous system (CNS) and exhibits an activated B cell phenotype by both immunohistochemistry and mutational analysis. Frequent alterations in *MYD88*, *CD79B*, and *CD274/PDCD1LG2* serve as valuable diagnostic and therapeutic biomarkers in this disease.

- Primary low-grade B cell lymphomas are a group of relatively indolent tumors that include extranodal marginal zone lymphoma (EMZL), lymphoplasmacytic lymphoma, and small lymphocytic lymphoma. Although little is currently known about their genomic signatures, use of molecular diagnostics can greatly facilitate accurate diagnosis.

- EMZL preferentially involves dura and can mimic meningioma clinically, rendering it particular amenable to surgical resection and radiotherapy.

- CNS T cell lymphomas are especially challenging diagnostically given their rarity and frequently banal histologic appearance. They usually demonstrate a CD8-positive cytotoxic phenotype, creating additional overlap with inflammatory conditions. As with B cell lymphoproliferative disorders, T cell lymphomas of the CNS show recurrent mutations that confirm the diagnosis of neoplasia and may guide therapeutic strategy.

ABSTRACT

Primary lymphoid neoplasms of the central nervous system are rare tumors that span a wide range of histopathologic appearances and can overlap occasionally with non-neoplastic processes. Application of modern molecular techniques has not only begun to unravel their unique underlying biology but has also started to lay a valuable diagnostic and therapeutic framework for these frequently aggressive malignancies. This review summarizes the existing landscape of clinicopathologic and genomic features of lymphoid neoplasms that may arise primarily within the central nervous system.

OVERVIEW

Primary lymphoid malignancies of the central nervous system (CNS) are a rare and diverse group of entities. The most common of these by far is primary diffuse large B cell lymphoma (DLBCL); however, low-grade B cell neoplasms and T cell lymphomas may be infrequently encountered and, thus, pose a significant challenge to the diagnostician. Despite the rarity of these neoplasms, recent work has begun to elucidate their genomic landscapes, providing not only new diagnostic biomarkers but also potential targets of therapy. This review summarizes both the clinicopathologic features of CNS lymphoid malignancies and

---

Department of Pathology, Brigham and Women's Hospital, Harvard Medical School, 75 Francis Street, Boston, MA 02115, USA
E-mail address: dmmeredith@bwh.harvard.edu

Surgical Pathology 13 (2020) 267–276
https://doi.org/10.1016/j.path.2020.02.001

recent trends in molecular diagnostics and treatment strategies.

DIFFUSE LARGE B CELL LYMPHOMA

Clinical Features

DLBCL of the CNS accounts for roughly 3% of all brain tumors and less than 1% of all non-Hodgkin lymphomas.[1] Although this lymphoma can arise in patients of any age, most cases occur between the fifth and seventh decades.[2,3] The supratentorial compartment is the most frequent site of involvement (60% of cases); however, the posterior fossa, leptomeninges, eye, and spinal cord may all be affected.[4] Tumors most often present as solitary lesions (60%–70% of cases), but multifocal disease may be encountered.[4] Although it is not uncommon for DLBCL arising in other sites to secondarily involve the CNS, primary CNS DLBCL very rarely recurs in extraneural locations.[5–8]

Epstein-Barr virus (EBV)-positive DLBCL occurs most frequently in the elderly, with a peak incidence in the eighth decade; however, there is a second smaller peak occurring in the third decade.[9,10] Although associated with immunodeficiency, as many as 5% to 15% of patients may have no predisposing conditions.[11–21]

Intravascular large B cell lymphoma (IVLBCL) is a rare form DLBCL having no solid organ primary that grows exclusively within small vessels. Although any organ may be affected, the CNS shows involvement in greater than 75% of cases.[22] IVLBCL preferentially occurs in older adults, with a median age of 67 years.[23–27]

Microscopy and Immunophenotype

Microscopically, DLBCL of the CNS is an infiltrative neoplasm that frequently exhibits sheeting and perivascular aggregates of tumor cells. Tumor cells show typical DLBCL morphology with high nuclear:cytoplasm ratio, coarse chromatin with one or more nucleoli, and frequent nuclear irregularity or clefting (Fig. 1A). Background brain tissue often shows marked reactive astrocytosis or frank necrosis, sometimes accompanied by a variably robust non-neoplastic lymphocytic infiltrate (Fig. 2) that may be mistaken for primary inflammatory disorders on small biopsy specimens. Importantly, tumors that have been treated with corticosteroids before biopsy may show little, if any, evidence of tumor involvement in an otherwise background of reactive brain tissue and lymphohistiocytic infiltrates.[28]

The tumor cells of IVLBCL closely resemble those in conventional CNS DLBCL, but are confined to vessel lumina with minimal extravasation into Virchow-Robin spaces and surrounding parenchyma. Importantly, the surrounding brain tissue often shows evidence of ischemic injury due to multifocal vascular occlusion, and careful examination must be conducted of the microvasculature for tumor cells, which can be present only focally.[28]

Immunohistochemistry in all forms of DLBCL demonstrates routine positivity for mature B cell markers, such as CD19, CD20, PAX5, and CD79a. Ki67 indices are exceptionally high, frequently exceeding 80% to 90%.[29] Over 80% of cases are double expressors of BCL2 (Fig. 1B) and MYC; unlike systemic DLBCL, however, this does not correspond well with translocation status, which is much rarer in the CNS.[29,30] Most cases exhibit an activated B cell phenotype and express BCL6 and MUM1 (Fig. 1C), whereas CD10 positivity is rare.[31] Overexpression of PD-L1 and PD-L2 may also be detected by immunohistochemistry; however, care must be taken to separate expression in background brain tissue and macrophages from infiltrating tumor cells (Fig. 1D).

EBV-driven tumors can be reliably classified by in situ hybridization for EBER.

Genetic Profile

CNS DLBCL shows a similar genetic profile to that of activated B cell (ABC) phenotype DLBCL elsewhere; however, the characteristic profile is much more stereotyped in the CNS. Activation of the Toll-like receptor, B cell receptor (BCR), and nuclear factor κB pathways are frequently observed, most often via activating mutations in MYD88 and CD79B and inactivating mutations in CARD11 and TNFAIP3.[32–41] Additional mutations in PIM1, TBL1XR1, IRF4, ETV6, and PRDM1 are also frequently encountered.[32,38–41]

Most CNS DLBCL demonstrate evidence of genomic instability and numerous copy-number alterations.[41] This is likely the result of frequent deletion of CDKN2A and/or FHIT, which occur far more often in CNS DLBCL than in ABC-type DLBCL elsewhere.[32,38,41] Additional commonly observed events include amplification of NFKBIZ on 3q12.3, gain of 18q (leading to BCL2 overexpression), and amplification of 9p24, including CD274 and PDCD1LG2.[41] Deletions of HLA class II genes on 6p21 are also seen in approximately 75% of CNS DLBCLs, further contributing to escape of immune surveillance.[32,37,41–43]

Structural variants involving BCL6 are considerably less common than in DLBCL arising outside the CNS, and rearrangements of MYC and BCL2 are essentially nonexistent.[29,41,44,45] Enhancer hijacking events leading to constitutive expression

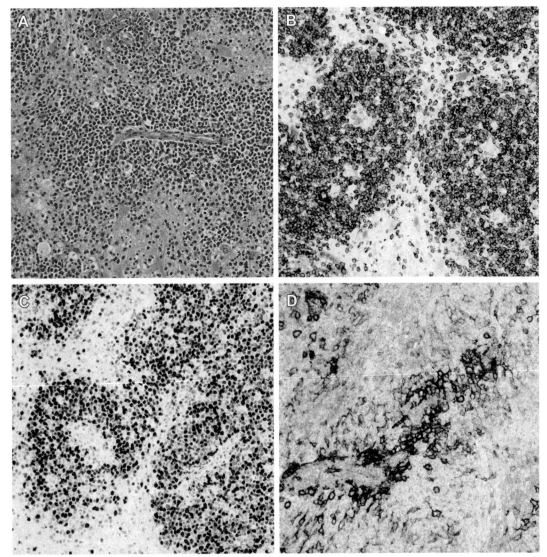

Fig. 1. Microscopic appearance of CNS DLBCL. (*A*) Tumor cells frequently aggregate around blood vessels and infiltrate into the surrounding brain parenchyma. Most CNS DLBCL exhibit increased expression of BCL2 (*B*) and MYC (not shown), along with the activated B cell markers MUM1 (*C*) and BCL6 (not shown). (*D*) PD-L1 immunopositivity can be patchy and correlates strongly with amplification or translocation of *CD274/PDCD1LG2*. Of note, infiltrating macrophages also show strong expression and must not be mistaken for tumor cells.

of PD-L1 and PD-L2 have been demonstrated in a small subset of cases.[41] Currently, RNA-based or custom-designed hybrid capture DNA sequencing platforms are required to detect these alterations; however, immunohistochemistry may be a reliable surrogate assay where available.[38,41]

In contrast, EBV-driven DLBCL shows few of the above alterations, with the exception of occasional gain of 9p24.[46,47]

Treatment Considerations

Until recently, the only viable options for treating CNS DLBCL were limited to high-dose chemotherapy regimens, usually including methotrexate, whole-brain radiation, and autologous stem cell transplant.[48] Although these agents show excellent short-term efficacy, most tumors will recur within 2 years, and as many as one-third of patients do not respond at all.[48–51] The discovery of highly recurrent, targetable alterations in CNS DLBCL has led to several promising studies showing improved survival with novel agents. The presence of 9p24 amplifications in a subset of tumors has spurred several studies to investigate the use of checkpoint inhibitors, although long-term efficacy remains to be determined.[52,53]

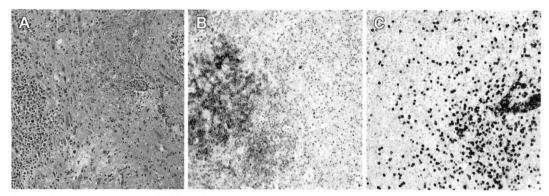

Fig. 2. Edge of DLBCL tumor. (*A*) Although most tumors show some degree of parenchymal infiltration, occasionally tumors show sharp boundaries with surrounding brain tissue with adjacent non-neoplastic inflammation and marked reactive changes. (*B*) CD20 highlights the tumor boundary, and CD3-positive T cells cluster in the adjacent reactive parenchyma (*C*).

Furthermore, early studies have begun to investigate the utility of BTK inhibition via ibrutinib, which has shown dramatic early results, even against tumors without evidence of *MYD88* or *CD79B* alterations.[54–56] Additional preclinical investigations have shown efficacy of targeted BCL2 and phosphoinositide 3-kinase (PI3K) inhibition in DLBCL models with evidence of BCR activation, which may soon be translated into clinical trials.[57]

Given the high rate of neurotoxicity associated with high-dose methotrexate and whole-brain radiation, targeted agents are likely to become first-line therapies in the near future, underscoring the importance of adequate tissue stewardship for molecular testing in this disease.

LOW-GRADE B CELL LYMPHOMAS

Clinical Features

Entities belonging to this broad category of lymphomas, including small lymphocytic lymphoma, extranodal marginal zone lymphoma (EMZL), follicular lymphoma, and lymphoplasmacytic lymphoma, arise primarily in the CNS with extreme rarity and account for less than 3% of all primary CNS lymphomas.[58,59] These lymphomas may occur throughout the CNS; however, the vast majority occur in the cerebral hemispheres.[60] EMZL by contrast shows a particular predilection for the dura, often forming mass lesions that can mimic meningioma.[61,62]

In addition, the histologic features of these tumors may be difficult to distinguish from inflammatory or infectious conditions, further leading to misdiagnosis. Ancillary molecular testing, therefore, can be of great utility in these cases.

Microscopy and Immunophenotype

The microscopic appearance of these lymphomas can vary somewhat, depending on the precise classification, but most cases generally contain dense or diffuse collections of small to medium lymphocytes with monomorphic to irregular nuclei and variable proportion of plasmacytoid forms (**Fig. 3**A). EMZL often forms a well-circumscribed mass lesion in the dura and may exhibit characteristic monocytoid forms, with clear cytoplasm and distinct cell borders (**Fig. 4**).[61] Perivascular collections may also be encountered. Cells are positive for CD20 and other mature B cell markers, and the plasma cell component shows monotypic light chain expression (**Fig. 3**B–E). CD5 and CD23 are generally negative outside of instances of small lymphocytic lymphoma. Ki67 proliferation rates are generally low (**Fig. 3**F).

Genetic Profile

Extensive analysis by fluorescence in situ hybridization of CNS marginal zone lymphomas showed no evidence of the characteristic translocations in *BCL6*, *MALT1*, or *IgH*.[61] Trisomy of chromosome 3 was the most common finding, followed by occasional polysomy of 7, 12, and 18.[61]

Although no published series exist to date describing the comprehensive mutational genomic signatures of low-grade CNS lymphomas, in this author's experience they tend to overlap with the expected signatures of similar extraneural examples. For example, mutations in *MYD88* would be most consistent with lymphoplasmacytic lymphoma, whereas evidence of NF-kB pathway activation via deletion of 6q23 (*TNFAIP3*) or another mechanism would suggest marginal zone origin.

Regardless, targeted sequencing panels can be of great utility in accurately subclassifying or confirming the diagnosis of neoplasia in these difficult cases, because immunoglobulin H (IgH) rearrangement studies do not always reveal clear

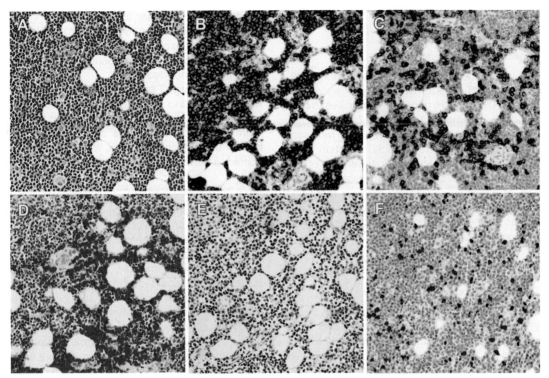

Fig. 3. Example of a low-grade B cell lymphoma involving a sacral nerve root with soft tissue extension. (*A*) The tumor is composed of small lymphocytes with minimal atypia and occasional plasmacytoid forms. (*B*) CD20 is diffusely positive in the lesion, and CD138 marks a subset of plasma cells (*C*). (*D*) The plasma cell component shows monotypic expression of kappa light chain by in situ hybridization compared with lambda light chain (*E*). (*F*) Ki67 staining demonstrates a low proliferative rate.

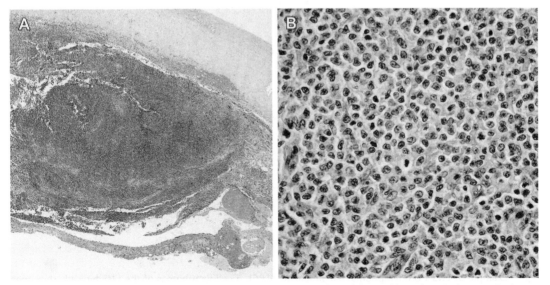

Fig. 4. Example of extranodal marginal zone lymphoma involving dura. (*A*) Dural-based EMZL frequently shows a circumscribed nodular pattern, which can mimic meningioma clinically. (*B*) High-power magnification of the tumor shows characteristic morphology with abundant clear cytoplasm ("monocytoid" appearance), distinct cell borders, irregular nuclei, and small nucleoli.

evidence of clonality, especially in the presence of dense background inflammation.

Treatment Considerations

As a group, these lymphomas are far more indolent than CNS DLBCL, with a 5-year survival of roughly 60%, and are generally responsive to conventional chemotherapeutic regimens.[59,63–68] Marginal zone lymphoma is particularly radiosensitive and amenable to surgical resection given its predilection for localized involvement of the dura, leading to complete remission in nearly 80% of patients.[62] Given the extreme rarity and hitherto lack of information regarding genomic profiles of these lesions, targeted therapy trials have not yet been attempted.

T CELL LYMPHOMAS

Clinical Features

Like low-grade B cell lymphomas, primary T cell lymphomas of the CNS are exquisitely rare, comprising fewer than 2% of all primary CNS lymphomas.[69,70] Incidence is higher is Asia than other parts of the world, and younger or middle-aged adults are preferentially affected.[59,71] All regions of the neuroaxis may be involved, with most examples arising in the cerebral hemispheres.[70,72] Most tumors are subclassified as peripheral T cell lymphoma when reported.[72]

Anaplastic large T cell lymphoma (ALCL) is even less common and tends to occur in children and young adults.[73–77] Involvement seems to be more prevalent in the dura and leptomeninges than in the CNS parenchyma, and ALK positivity confers a better prognosis.[74]

Microscopy and Immunophenotype

T cell lymphomas may exhibit a wide spectrum of morphologies, and definitive diagnosis usually requires demonstrating aberrant T cell immunophenotype or evidence of clonality. Tumor cells are generally small to medium sized with irregular nuclei, finely dispersed chromatin, and variably prominent nucleoli.[28,72] Similar to CNS DLBCL, CNS T cell lymphomas often show dense clustering around blood vessels and background necrosis (**Fig. 5**A). Diffuse parenchymal infiltration is also commonly observed, which can prove especially challenging diagnostically on small biopsies

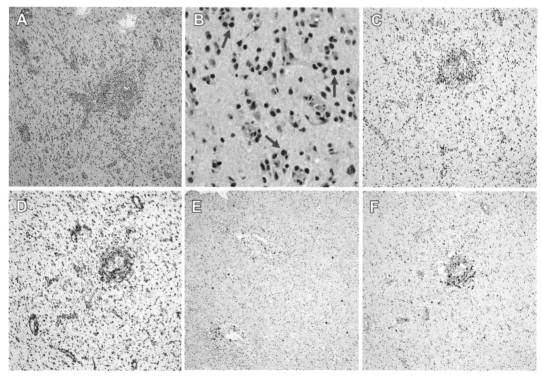

Fig. 5. Example of CNS T cell lymphoma. (*A*) Similar to DLBCL, T cell lymphomas of the CNS typically show perivascular aggregates of tumor cells that diffusely infiltrate surrounding brain tissue. (*B*) Higher magnification of the infiltrating component illustrates the subtlety that these lesions may exhibit, with intermediate-sized cells showing minimal atypia and nuclear hyperchromasia (*arrows*). This tumor expressed CD3 (*C*) and showed subset loss of CD2 (*F*). Uncharacteristically, this example showed CD4 positivity (*D*) and was negative for CD8 (*E*).

(Fig. 5B). Large-cell variants may mimic DLBCL morphologically and contain characteristic "hallmark" cells.[72]

Most tumors show loss of one or more of the T cell markers CD2, CD3, CD5, and CD7 (Fig. 5C and F).[28,72] A cytotoxic CD8-positive phenotype is common irrespective of morphology, and positivity for TIA1, granzyme-B, and perforin can lead to confusion with inflammatory conditions.[28,72] Less often, CD4-positive or aberrant double-negative (CD4–/CD8–) phenotypes may be observed (Fig. 5D and E).[72] ALCL also shows typical expression of CD30 and ALK.[72]

Genetic Profile

Irrespective of microscopic appearance, evidence of T cell receptor clonality is almost universal.[72] Genomic evaluation of CNS T cell lymphomas has been quite limited to date, with targeted sequencing data available for only a handful of cases. Nonetheless, mutations in commonly implicated genes in other T cell lymphomas, such as DNMT3A, GNB1, KRAS, TET2, JAK3, STAT3, and STAT5B have been reported.[72]

Treatment Consideration

Prognosis for primary CNS T cell lymphoma is generally poor with few long-term survivors. Median survival for patients has been reported at 25 months, and 1 study of 7 patients showed similar outcomes relative to patients with CNS DLBCL.[59,70] Although there is no consensus as to optimal treatment regimen, most include high-dose methotrexate followed by autologous stem cell transplantation.[70,78]

Nonetheless, several targeted approaches are being explored in systemic T cell malignancies that may show benefit in CNS tumors. Federal Drug Administration approval already exists for use of the anti-CD30 antibody-drug conjugate brentuximab vedotin in CD30-positive lymphomas and the ALK inhibitor crizotinib in ALK-positive ALCL.[79,80] Furthermore, several clinical trials have already opened exploring the efficacy of other targeted regimens against commonly activated pathways in T cell lymphoma, including inhibitors against PI3K, Jak/STAT signaling, and DNA methylation.[80]

SUMMARY

DLBCL is by far the most common primary lymphoid malignancy of the CNS and, given adequate tissue sampling, is rarely a diagnostic conundrum. Nonetheless, molecular studies have identified a stereotyped genomic signature in CNS DLBCL that implicates a distinct biology from extraneural examples and provides a rich array of druggable targets. Less common neoplasms, including T cell lymphomas and low-grade B cell lymphomas, may pose a much greater diagnostic challenge and overlap considerably with inflammatory or infectious processes. Here again, ancillary molecular testing can solidify the diagnosis of neoplasia, assist with subclassification, and help direct treatment. As neuropathology continues to move toward routine molecular testing for classifying and identifying clinically relevant biomarkers in brain tumors, lymphoid neoplasms are also likely to benefit from this approach, and proper conservation and triage of tissue should be considered in the handling of these cases.

DISCLOSURE

The authors have nothing to disclose.

REFERENCES

1. Schlegel U. Primary CNS lymphoma. Ther Adv Neurol Disord 2009;2(2):93–104.
2. Cote TR, Manns A, Hardy CR, et al. Epidemiology of brain lymphoma among people with or without acquired immunodeficiency syndrome. AIDS/Cancer Study Group. J Natl Cancer Inst 1996;88(10):675–9.
3. Villano JL, Koshy M, Shaikh H, et al. Age, gender, and racial differences in incidence and survival in primary CNS lymphoma. Br J Cancer 2011;105(9):1414–8.
4. Deckert M, Engert A, Bruck W, et al. Modern concepts in the biology, diagnosis, differential diagnosis and treatment of primary central nervous system lymphoma. Leukemia 2011;25(12):1797–807.
5. Booman M, Douwes J, Legdeur MC, et al. From brain to testis: immune escape and clonal selection in a B cell lymphoma with selective outgrowth in two immune sanctuaries. Haematologica 2007;92(6):e69–71.
6. Harney J, Pope A, Short SC. Primary central nervous system lymphoma with testicular relapse. Clin Oncol (R Coll Radiol) 2004;16(3):193–5.
7. Jahnke K, Thiel E, Martus P, et al. Relapse of primary central nervous system lymphoma: clinical features, outcome and prognostic factors. J Neurooncol 2006;80(2):159–65.
8. Rajappa SJ, Uppin SG, Digumarti R. Testicular relapse of primary central nervous system lymphoma. Leuk Lymphoma 2007;48(5):1023–5.
9. Nicolae A, Pittaluga S, Abdullah S, et al. EBV-positive large-B-cell lymphomas in young patients: a nodal lymphoma with evidence for a tolerogenic immune environment. Blood 2015;126(7):863–72.

10. Shimoyama Y, Yamamoto K, Asano N, et al. Age-related Epstein-Barr virus-associated B-cell lymphoproliferative disorders: special references to lymphomas surrounding this newly recognized clinicopathologic disease. Cancer Sci 2008;99(6): 1085–91.

11. Beltran BE, Castillo JJ, Morales D, et al. EBV-positive diffuse large B-cell lymphoma of the elderly: a case series from Peru. Am J Hematol 2011;86(8):663–7.

12. Dojcinov SD, Venkataraman G, Pittaluga S, et al. Age-related EBV-associated lymphoproliferative disorders in the Western population: a spectrum of reactive lymphoid hyperplasia and lymphoma. Blood 2011;117(18):4726–35.

13. Gibson SE, Hsi ED. Epstein-Barr virus-positive B-cell lymphoma of the elderly at a United States tertiary medical center: an uncommon aggressive lymphoma with a nongerminal center B-cell phenotype. Hum Pathol 2009;40(5):653–61.

14. Hong JY, Ko YH, Kim SJ, et al. Epstein-Barr virus-positive diffuse large B-cell lymphoma of the elderly: a concise review and update. Curr Opin Oncol 2015; 27(5):392–8.

15. Lu TX, Liang JH, Miao Y, et al. Epstein-Barr virus positive diffuse large B-cell lymphoma predict poor outcome, regardless of the age. Sci Rep 2015;5: 12168.

16. Montes-Moreno S, Odqvist L, Diaz-Perez JA, et al. EBV-positive diffuse large B-cell lymphoma of the elderly is an aggressive post-germinal center B-cell neoplasm characterized by prominent nuclear factor-kB activation. Mod Pathol 2012;25(7):968–82.

17. Ok CY, Li L, Xu-Monette ZY, et al. Prevalence and clinical implications of Epstein-Barr virus infection in de novo diffuse large B-cell lymphoma in Western countries. Clin Cancer Res 2014;20(9):2338–49.

18. Ok CY, Papathomas TG, Medeiros LJ, et al. EBV-positive diffuse large B-cell lymphoma of the elderly. Blood 2013;122(3):328–40.

19. Oyama T, Ichimura K, Suzuki R, et al. Senile EBV+ B-cell lymphoproliferative disorders: a clinicopathologic study of 22 patients. Am J Surg Pathol 2003; 27(1):16–26.

20. Oyama T, Yamamoto K, Asano N, et al. Age-related EBV-associated B-cell lymphoproliferative disorders constitute a distinct clinicopathologic group: a study of 96 patients. Clin Cancer Res 2007;13(17): 5124–32.

21. Park S, Lee J, Ko YH, et al. The impact of Epstein-Barr virus status on clinical outcome in diffuse large B-cell lymphoma. Blood 2007;110(3):972–8.

22. Beristain X, Azzarelli B. The neurological masquerade of intravascular lymphomatosis. Arch Neurol 2002;59(3):439–43.

23. Ferreri AJ, Dognini GP, Campo E, et al. Variations in clinical presentation, frequency of hemophagocytosis and clinical behavior of intravascular lymphoma diagnosed in different geographical regions. Haematologica 2007;92(4):486–92.

24. Murase T, Yamaguchi M, Suzuki R, et al. Intravascular large B-cell lymphoma (IVLBCL): a clinicopathologic study of 96 cases with special reference to the immunophenotypic heterogeneity of CD5. Blood 2007;109(2):478–85.

25. Ponzoni M, Ferreri AJ. Intravascular lymphoma: a neoplasm of 'homeless' lymphocytes? Hematol Oncol 2006;24(3):105–12.

26. Ponzoni M, Ferreri AJ, Campo E, et al. Definition, diagnosis, and management of intravascular large B-cell lymphoma: proposals and perspectives from an international consensus meeting. J Clin Oncol 2007;25(21):3168–73.

27. Shimada K, Kinoshita T, Naoe T, et al. Presentation and management of intravascular large B-cell lymphoma. Lancet Oncol 2009;10(9):895–902.

28. Giannini C, Dogan A, Salomao DR. CNS lymphoma: a practical diagnostic approach. J Neuropathol Exp Neurol 2014;73(6):478–94.

29. Brunn A, Nagel I, Montesinos-Rongen M, et al. Frequent triple-hit expression of MYC, BCL2, and BCL6 in primary lymphoma of the central nervous system and absence of a favorable MYC(low)BCL2 (low) subgroup may underlie the inferior prognosis as compared to systemic diffuse large B cell lymphomas. Acta Neuropathol 2013;126(4):603–5.

30. Cobbers JM, Wolter M, Reifenberger J, et al. Frequent inactivation of CDKN2A and rare mutation of TP53 in PCNSL. Brain Pathol 1998;8(2):263–76.

31. Deckert M, Brunn A, Montesinos-Rongen M, et al. Primary lymphoma of the central nervous system— a diagnostic challenge. Hematol Oncol 2014;32(2): 57–67.

32. Gonzalez-Aguilar A, Idbaih A, Boisselier B, et al. Recurrent mutations of MYD88 and TBL1XR1 in primary central nervous system lymphomas. Clin Cancer Res 2012;18(19):5203–11.

33. Kraan W, Horlings HM, van Keimpema M, et al. High prevalence of oncogenic MYD88 and CD79B mutations in diffuse large B-cell lymphomas presenting at immune-privileged sites. Blood Cancer J 2013;3: e139.

34. Montesinos-Rongen M, Godlewska E, Brunn A, et al. Activating L265P mutations of the MYD88 gene are common in primary central nervous system lymphoma. Acta Neuropathol 2011;122(6):791–2.

35. Montesinos-Rongen M, Schmitz R, Brunn A, et al. Mutations of CARD11 but not TNFAIP3 may activate the NF-kappaB pathway in primary CNS lymphoma. Acta Neuropathol 2010;120(4):529–35.

36. Montesinos-Rongen M, Schafer E, Siebert R, et al. Genes regulating the B cell receptor pathway are recurrently mutated in primary central nervous system lymphoma. Acta Neuropathol 2012;124(6): 905–6.

37. Schwindt H, Vater I, Kreuz M, et al. Chromosomal imbalances and partial uniparental disomies in primary central nervous system lymphoma. Leukemia 2009;23(10):1875–84.

38. Nayyar N, White MD, Gill CM, et al. MYD88 L265P mutation and CDKN2A loss are early mutational events in primary central nervous system diffuse large B-cell lymphomas. Blood Adv 2019;3(3):375–83.

39. Bruno A, Boisselier B, Labreche K, et al. Mutational analysis of primary central nervous system lymphoma. Oncotarget 2014;5(13):5065–75.

40. Vater I, Montesinos-Rongen M, Schlesner M, et al. The mutational pattern of primary lymphoma of the central nervous system determined by whole-exome sequencing. Leukemia 2015;29(3):677–85.

41. Chapuy B, Roemer MG, Stewart C, et al. Targetable genetic features of primary testicular and primary central nervous system lymphomas. Blood 2016; 127(7):869–81.

42. Jordanova ES, Riemersma SA, Philippo K, et al. Hemizygous deletions in the HLA region account for loss of heterozygosity in the majority of diffuse large B-cell lymphomas of the testis and the central nervous system. Genes Chromosomes Cancer 2002;35(1):38–48.

43. Riemersma SA, Jordanova ES, Schop RF, et al. Extensive genetic alterations of the HLA region, including homozygous deletions of HLA class II genes in B-cell lymphomas arising in immune-privileged sites. Blood 2000;96(10):3569–77.

44. Cady FM, O'Neill BP, Law ME, et al. Del(6)(q22) and BCL6 rearrangements in primary CNS lymphoma are indicators of an aggressive clinical course. J Clin Oncol 2008;26(29):4814–9.

45. Montesinos-Rongen M, Zuhlke-Jenisch R, Gesk S, et al. Interphase cytogenetic analysis of lymphoma-associated chromosomal breakpoints in primary diffuse large B-cell lymphomas of the central nervous system. J Neuropathol Exp Neurol 2002;61(10):926–33.

46. Gebauer N, Gebauer J, Hardel TT, et al. Prevalence of targetable oncogenic mutations and genomic alterations in Epstein-Barr virus-associated diffuse large B-cell lymphoma of the elderly. Leuk Lymphoma 2015;56(4):1100–6.

47. Yoon H, Park S, Ju H, et al. Integrated copy number and gene expression profiling analysis of Epstein-Barr virus-positive diffuse large B-cell lymphoma. Genes Chromosomes Cancer 2015;54(6):383–96.

48. Nayak L, Batchelor TT. Recent advances in treatment of primary central nervous system lymphoma. Curr Treat Options Oncol 2013;14(4):539–52.

49. Korfel A, Schlegel U. Diagnosis and treatment of primary CNS lymphoma. Nat Rev Neurol 2013;9(6):317–27.

50. Hoang-Xuan K, Bessell E, Bromberg J, et al. Diagnosis and treatment of primary CNS lymphoma in immunocompetent patients: guidelines from the European Association for Neuro-Oncology. Lancet Oncol 2015;16(7):e322–32.

51. Langner-Lemercier S, Houillier C, Soussain C, et al. Primary CNS lymphoma at first relapse/progression: characteristics, management, and outcome of 256 patients from the French LOC network. Neuro Oncol 2016;18(9):1297–303.

52. Nayak L, Iwamoto FM, LaCasce A, et al. PD-1 blockade with nivolumab in relapsed/refractory primary central nervous system and testicular lymphoma. Blood 2017;129(23):3071–3.

53. Grommes C, Nayak L, Tun HW, et al. Introduction of novel agents in the treatment of primary CNS lymphoma. Neuro Oncol 2019;21(3):306–13.

54. Grommes C, Pastore A, Palaskas N, et al. Ibrutinib unmasks critical role of Bruton tyrosine kinase in primary CNS lymphoma. Cancer Discov 2017;7(9):1018–29.

55. Lionakis MS, Dunleavy K, Roschewski M, et al. Inhibition of B cell receptor signaling by ibrutinib in primary CNS lymphoma. Cancer Cell 2017;31(6):833–43.e5.

56. Soussain C, Choquet S, Blonski M, et al. Ibrutinib monotherapy for relapse or refractory primary CNS lymphoma and primary vitreoretinal lymphoma: final analysis of the phase II 'proof-of-concept' iLOC study by the Lymphoma Study Association (LYSA) and the French oculo-cerebral lymphoma (LOC) network. Eur J Cancer 2019;117:121–30.

57. Bojarczuk K, Wienand K, Ryan JA, et al. Targeted inhibition of PI3Kalpha/delta is synergistic with BCL-2 blockade in genetically defined subtypes of DLBCL. Blood 2019;133(1):70–80.

58. Jahnke K, Thiel E, Schilling A, et al. Low-grade primary central nervous system lymphoma in immunocompetent patients. Br J Haematol 2005;128(5):616–24.

59. Lim T, Kim SJ, Kim K, et al. Primary CNS lymphoma other than DLBCL: a descriptive analysis of clinical features and treatment outcomes. Ann Hematol 2011;90(12):1391–8.

60. Jahnke K, Korfel A, O'Neill BP, et al. International study on low-grade primary central nervous system lymphoma. Ann Neurol 2006;59(5):755–62.

61. Tu PH, Giannini C, Judkins AR, et al. Clinicopathologic and genetic profile of intracranial marginal zone lymphoma: a primary low-grade CNS lymphoma that mimics meningioma. J Clin Oncol 2005;23(24):5718–27.

62. Ayanambakkam A, Ibrahimi S, Bilal K, et al. Extranodal marginal zone lymphoma of the central nervous system. Clin Lymphoma Myeloma Leuk 2018;18(1):34–7.e8.

63. Aziz M, Chaurasia JK, Khan R, et al. Primary low-grade diffuse small lymphocytic lymphoma of the central nervous system. BMJ Case Rep 2014;2014.

64. Papanicolau-Sengos A, Wang-Rodriguez J, Wang HY, et al. Rare case of a primary non-dural central nervous system low grade B-cell lymphoma and literature review. Int J Clin Exp Pathol 2012;5(1):89–95.

65. Ponzoni M, Bonetti F, Poliani PL, et al. Central nervous system marginal zone B-cell lymphoma associated with *Chlamydophila psittaci* infection. Hum Pathol 2011;42(5):738–42.

66. Schiefer AI, Vastagh I, Molnar MJ, et al. Extranodal marginal zone lymphoma of the CNS arising after a long-standing history of atypical white matter disease. Leuk Res 2012;36(7):e155–7.

67. Skardelly M, Pantazis G, Bisdas S, et al. Primary cerebral low-grade B-cell lymphoma, monoclonal immunoglobulin deposition disease, cerebral light chain deposition disease and "aggregoma": an update on classification and diagnosis. BMC Neurol 2013;13:107.

68. Ueba T, Okawa M, Abe H, et al. Central nervous system marginal zone B-cell lymphoma of mucosa-associated lymphoid tissue type involving the brain and spinal cord parenchyma. Neuropathology 2013;33(3):306–11.

69. Ferreri AJ, Reni M, Pasini F, et al. A multicenter study of treatment of primary CNS lymphoma. Neurology 2002;58(10):1513–20.

70. Shenkier TN, Blay JY, O'Neill BP, et al. Primary CNS lymphoma of T-cell origin: a descriptive analysis from the international primary CNS lymphoma collaborative group. J Clin Oncol 2005;23(10):2233–9.

71. Choi JS, Nam DH, Ko YH, et al. Primary central nervous system lymphoma in Korea: comparison of B- and T-cell lymphomas. Am J Surg Pathol 2003; 27(7):919–28.

72. Menon MP, Nicolae A, Meeker H, et al. Primary CNS T-cell lymphomas: a clinical, morphologic, immunophenotypic, and molecular analysis. Am J Surg Pathol 2015;39(12):1719–29.

73. Furuya K, Takanashi S, Ogawa A, et al. High-dose methotrexate monotherapy followed by radiation for CD30-positive, anaplastic lymphoma kinase-1-positive anaplastic large-cell lymphoma in the brain of a child. J Neurosurg Pediatr 2014;14(3):311–5.

74. George DH, Scheithauer BW, Aker FV, et al. Primary anaplastic large cell lymphoma of the central nervous system: prognostic effect of ALK-1 expression. Am J Surg Pathol 2003;27(4):487–93.

75. Merlin E, Chabrier S, Verkarre V, et al. Primary leptomeningeal ALK+ lymphoma in a 13-year-old child. J Pediatr Hematol Oncol 2008;30(12):963–7.

76. Park JS, Park H, Park S, et al. Primary central nervous system ALK positive anaplastic large cell lymphoma with predominantly leptomeningeal involvement in an adult. Yonsei Med J 2013;54(3): 791–6.

77. Vivekanandan S, Dickinson P, Bessell E, et al. An unusual case of primary anaplastic large cell central nervous system lymphoma: an 8-year success story. BMJ Case Rep 2011;2011, [pii:bcr1120103550].

78. Chihara D, Oki Y. Central nervous system involvement in peripheral T cell lymphoma. Curr Hematol Malig Rep 2018;13(1):1–6.

79. Foyil KV, Bartlett NL. Brentuximab vedotin and crizotinib in anaplastic large-cell lymphoma. Cancer J 2012;18(5):450–6.

80. Ng SY, Jacobsen ED. Peripheral T-cell lymphoma: moving toward targeted therapies. Hematol Oncol Clin North Am 2019;33(4):657–68.

Molecular and Histologic Diagnosis of Central Nervous System Infections

Isaac H. Solomon, MD, PhD

KEYWORDS

- Meningitis • Encephalitis • 16S rRNA • Internal transcribed spacer
- Metagenomic next-generation sequencing

Key points

- A wide range of microorganisms, including bacteria, mycobacteria, fungi, viruses, and parasites, can infect the central nervous system and cause significant morbidity and mortality.

- Diagnosis of CNS infections from surgical biopsies requires integration of histologic findings, including special stains and immunohistochemistry, with cultures, molecular diagnostics, and other laboratory and clinical findings.

- Molecular diagnostics performed on formalin-fixed paraffin-embedded tissue can be targeted at individual pathogens, classes of microorganisms, panels of organisms, or be completely unbiased.

ABSTRACT

Infections of the central nervous system cause significant morbidity and mortality in immunocompetent and immunocompromised individuals. A wide variety of microorganisms can cause infections, including bacteria, mycobacteria, fungi, viruses, and parasites. Although less invasive testing is preferred, surgical biopsy may be necessary to collect diagnostic tissue. Histologic findings, including special stains and immunohistochemistry, can provide a morphologic diagnosis in many cases, which can be further classified by molecular testing. Correlation of molecular, culture, and other laboratory results with histologic findings is essential for an accurate diagnosis, and to minimize false positives from microbial contamination.

OVERVIEW

The central nervous system (CNS) can be infected by a variety of microorganisms, resulting in significant morbidity and mortality. A variety of bacteria, mycobacteria, fungi, viruses, and parasites have been reported to cause disease, with significant variations in incidence associated with geography, age, and immune status. Some highly virulent pathogens cause disease in otherwise healthy individuals, whereas many others opportunistically infect people with compromised immune systems. People living with human immunodeficiency virus (HIV), organ transplant recipients, immunotherapy-treated individuals, and infants and the elderly are all at increased risk for a variety of infections. The most common route of CNS infection is hematogenous, with symptoms that are predominantly neurologic or manifest as part of a disseminated systemic disease. Infections can also be spread by local extension from adjacent structures (eg, paranasal sinuses), retrograde axonal transport, and introduced by trauma or surgery. Symptoms, which can range from mild headaches to herniation and death, depend on the specific areas of brain or spinal cord involved, acuity of the infection, and any prior immunity acquired by the patient.

Diagnosis of CNS infections largely relies on testing performed in the clinical laboratories. Examination of cerebrospinal fluid (CSF) collected via lumbar puncture can provide insight into

Department of Pathology, Brigham and Women's Hospital, Harvard Medical School, 75 Francis Street, Boston, MA 02115, USA
E-mail address: ihsolomon@bwh.harvard.edu

Surgical Pathology 13 (2020) 277–289
https://doi.org/10.1016/j.path.2020.01.001
1875-9181/20/© 2020 Elsevier Inc. All rights reserved.

surgpath.theclinics.com

possible infectious etiologies based on opening pressure, color, protein, glucose, and cell counts. Further testing including cultures, serology, and molecular diagnostics can identify specific microorganisms, which is critical for the selection of appropriate antimicrobial therapy. When less invasive testing is nondiagnostic, surgical sampling of brain or spinal cord tissue is performed, either as a core biopsy, or as a larger resection in conjunction with efforts to relieve elevations of intracranial pressure. Standard histopathologic evaluation of tissue, including special stains, can provide a great deal of information about infections through identification of characteristic inflammatory patterns and by direct visualization of organisms. Further characterization is achieved by immunohistochemistry and the selective use of targeted and broad-spectrum molecular assays. This review highlights the utility of molecular testing for the diagnosis of CNS infections, presents recommendations for histologic screening to guide molecular assay selection, and suggests

strategies for integration of unexpected molecular findings (**Table 1**). Although several examples are discussed, a comprehensive list of diagnostic features for all possible CNS infections is beyond the scope of this article, and consultation with infectious disease textbooks or pathologists is recommended.[1–3]

BACTERIAL INFECTIONS

EPIDEMIOLOGY AND LABORATORY DIAGNOSTICS

Bacterial meningitis is the most common CNS infection, and affects 0.7 to 40 per 100,000 people per year depending on geographic location.[4] In the absence of vaccination, Group B *Streptococcus*, *Streptococcus pneumoniae*, *Listeria monocytogenes*, *Escherichia coli*, *Neisseria meningitides*, and *Haemophilus influenza* are the most commonly identified organisms with varying frequency from newborns to young adults.

Table 1
Overview of histologic features and broad-spectrum molecular assays for diagnosis of CNS infections

Organism	H&E	Special Stains	Immunohistochemistry	Molecular Assays
Bacteria	Cocci and bacilli variably visible	Gram, Warthin-Starry, Steiner, PAS (*Tropheryma whipplei*)	*Treponema*	16S rRNA
Mycobacteria	Rarely detectable	Ziehl-Neelsen, Fite-Faraco	Not widely used	16S rRNA, *hsp65*, *rpoB*, IS6110 (*Mycobacterium tuberculosis*)
Fungi	Yeast and hyphae often visible as eosinophilic or negatively staining structures	GMS, PAS, Gram (*Candida*), Mucicarmine/Fontana-Masson (*Cryptococcus*)	Not widely used	28S rRNA D1/D2, ITS
Viruses	Characteristic cytoplasmic or nuclear inclusions present for some viruses	Luxol fast blue (PML)	HSV, VZV, EBV (ISH), CMV, adenovirus, polyomavirus	mNGS
Parasites	Diagnosis based predominantly on morphologic features	Giemsa, acid fast (cestode hooklets), GMS/PAS (ameba cyst walls)	*Toxoplasma*	mNGS

Abbreviations: CMV, cytomegalovirus; EBV, Epstein-Barr virus; GMS, Grocott-Gomori methenamine–silver nitrate stain; H&E, hematoxylin and eosin; HSV, herpes simplex virus; ISH, in situ hybridization; ITS, internal transcribed spacer; mNGS, metagenomic next-generation sequencing; PAS, periodic acid–Schiff; PML, progressive multifocal leukoencephalopathy; VZV, varicella zoster virus.

Parenchymal involvement, most often as cerebral abscess or cerebritis, is caused by *Staphylococcus aureus*, *Streptococcus* spp., Enterobacteriaceae, anaerobes, and may be polymicrobial.[5] CSF or brain tissue cultures are typically the test of choice for diagnosis, allowing for species-level identification and phenotypic information on antibiotic susceptibilities. The recent integration of matrix-assisted laser desorption/ionization time-of-flight mass spectrometry into routine clinical laboratory use has markedly improved the accuracy and speed of diagnosis once an organism has been isolated, and assays to directly test CSF are currently under development.[6] In addition, individual organisms or panels of common pathogens can be selectively targeted for rapid diagnosis (eg, Biofire ME panel, Salt Lake City, Utah).[7]

HISTOLOGIC FEATURES

Compared with autopsy series, surgical tissue is rarely obtained for the diagnosis of bacterial meningitis. Characteristic histologic features include abundant neutrophilic infiltration of the leptomeninges, and infarction of cortex because of compromised blood flow through surface vessels may be present. Abscess tissue may be collected during surgery to relieve intracranial pressure caused by mass effect, and to rule out neoplastic processes or other noninfectious etiologies. Lesions vary from millimeter-sized microabscesses to multi-centimeter-sized lesions. A necrotic center is typically surrounded by a rim of neutrophils and dying tissue, although inflammation may be limited in immunocompromised patients (**Fig. 1**A). Early lesions may only show neutrophilic inflammation in the form of cerebritis, which may be biopsied to diagnose a radiologic abnormality.[8] Depending on the acuity of the infection and extent of preceding antibiotic treatment, organisms may not be observed, even in the setting of positive cultures or molecular testing. Some bacteria (cocci and bacilli) are seen on routine hematoxylin and eosin (H&E) stains as eosinophilic or basophilic structures, but must be distinguished from necrosis and apoptotic debris. Gram-positive organisms including staphylococci and streptococci are best visualized with tissue Gram stains, such as Brown-Brenn and Lillie-Twort, which can also highlight Gram-negative organisms with varying success (**Fig. 1**B). Silver stains including Warthin-Starry and Steiner can identify a wide variety of organisms, but are particularly useful for Gram-negatives and spirochetes (**Fig. 1**C). Grocott-Gomori methenamine–silver nitrate stain (GMS), primarily used to identify fungi, can also stain bacteria, including Gram-positive organisms that have

stained Gram-negative because of antibiotic treatment effects. Periodic acid–Schiff (PAS) can highlight *Tropheryma whipplei* bacilli within macrophages. Although numerous antibodies for bacteria are available, the large degree of cross-reactivity between species and genera limits widespread adoption because of limited clinical utility. One notable exception is antitreponemal antibodies for the diagnosis of syphilis and other spirochete-associated diseases with increased sensitivity compared with silver stains.[9] *In situ* hybridization for the bacterial 16S rRNA gene has been investigated as a research tool, but not yet implemented as a diagnostic test for CNS bacterial infections.[10] Morphologic descriptions including shape, Gram status, and arrangement (eg, Gram-negative diplococci) can help guide empiric antibiotic therapy, and should be correlated with available culture and molecular results (eg, morphologically compatible with *N. meningitides* isolated in culture). Given the frequency of polymicrobial or multiple concurrent infections, caution should be used in making definitive statements regarding organism identifications in most circumstances.

MOLECULAR DIAGNOSTICS

When cultures are negative or not attempted, molecular testing of formalin-fixed paraffin-embedded (FFPE) tissue is performed to identify potential pathogens including bacteria. Unless a specific organism is suspected, the broad range test of choice is sequencing of the 16S rRNA gene, an approximately 1500 base pair gene that contains multiple conserved and variable regions useful for phylogenetic classification and clinical diagnosis.[11] Although sequencing the full gene produces the greatest amount of information, this is difficult to achieve in formalin-treated tissue because of DNA fragmentation and shorter reads.[12] A large proportion of pathogenic species are distinguished by sequencing the V1 and V2 regions consisting of an approximately 250 base pair sequence.[13] Clinical and Laboratory Standards Institute guidelines have been developed for genus and species identifications made by 16S sequencing, which specify percentage agreement with reference sequences and difference from next closest species (eg, 98.5% with 1.0% to next closest species).[14] False positives with 16S sequencing may occur because of contamination at multiple points in the gross pathology, histology, and molecular laboratories.[15] Therefore, extreme caution should be used in interpreting molecular results of unusual organisms, particularly when there is a discrepancy with histologic findings. All such cases should be rereviewed,

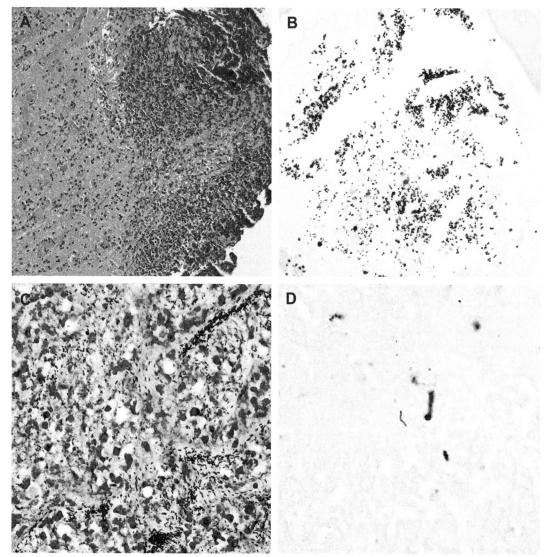

Fig. 1. Bacterial and mycobacterial infections. (*A*) This frontal lobe biopsy shows brain with reactive changes and abscess formation, findings suggestive of an infectious process. Correlation with special stains, concurrent culture results, or testing by 16S rRNA gene sequencing is necessary for confirmation and further classification of a bacterial infection (hematoxylin-eosin, original magnification ×200x). (*B*) Gram stain (original magnification ×400x) of a bone flap from a prior craniotomy highlights clusters of Gram-positive cocci, morphologically compatible with *Staphylococcus aureus* isolated in culture. (*C*) Warthin-Starry stain (original magnification ×400x) of subdural material shows multiple bacilli that are negative on Gram stain (not shown), morphologically compatible with *Pseudomonas aeruginosa* isolated in culture. (*D*) Ziehl-Neelsen staining (original magnification ×1000x) of a right frontal dural-based mass with necrotizing granulomas highlights rare acid-fast bacilli, consistent with *Mycobacterium tuberculosis*.

and an interpretative comment stating the possibility of contamination is added in an addendum (eg, the molecular findings of *Meiothermus silvanus* [a Gram-negative bacillus] is discordant with the presence of Gram-positive cocci observed histologically, raising the possibility of a false-positive molecular finding caused by laboratory contamination).

MYCOBACTERIAL INFECTIONS

EPIDEMIOLOGY AND LABORATORY DIAGNOSTICS

Mycobacterial infections of the CNS are typically caused by *Mycobacterium tuberculosis*, which can manifest as tuberculous meningitis, tuberculoma, or abscess.[16] Less commonly, non-tuberculous mycobacteria (NTM) is involved, and *Mycobacterium bovis* bacillus Calmette-Guérin vaccine strain is a rare cause of disseminated disease.[17] *Mycobacterium leprae* affects peripheral nerves, but has not been reported to have a significant impact on the CNS.[18] Many *Mycobacterium* spp. are slow-growing, taking weeks to months for culture isolation from CSF or brain tissue.[19] Treatment typically requires greater than 6 months with multiple antibiotics, which is determined empirically by species identification or through phenotypic testing.[20] CNS involvement, although rare, can often be suspected in the setting of active pulmonary or disseminated disease, which is rapidly diagnosed by polymerase chain reaction (PCR) of sputum, bronchoalveolar lavage fluid, or other tissue samples.[21]

HISTOLOGIC FEATURES

Biopsies of dural-based or parenchymal lesions typically show necrotizing granulomas, comprised of a necrotic center surrounded by a rim of multinucleated giant cells, lymphocytes, and plasma cells. Lesions early in development may show a neutrophilic predominance. Some NTMs exhibit a large number of histiocytes containing numerous organisms. The presence of mycobacteria is demonstrated by acid-fast staining methods, such as Ziehl-Neelsen and Fite-Faraco, in which carbol fuchsin is retained in the cell walls after acid decolorization (**Fig.** 1D). Although mycobacteria show some variations in length and width, these features, particularly in tissue sections that contain transected organisms, are not reliable for speciation. Mycobacterial immunostains are commercially available, but have limited specificity and must be interpreted in the appropriate histopathologic context.[22] Partially acid-fast organisms including *Nocarida* spp. can also stain with modified acid-fast stains, a distinguishing feature from *Actinomyces* spp., both of which are filamentous Gram-positive bacteria that are detected by Gram and GMS stains.

MOLECULAR DIAGNOSTICS

Because of the slow-growing nature of many mycobacteria, molecular testing of FFPE has been used to provide a more rapid species-level diagnosis to help guide antibiotic therapy. Similar to other bacteria, 16S rRNA sequencing is used to distinguish many *Mycobacterium* spp. Additional targets with increased interspecies variability include *heat shock protein 65* (*hsp65*) and beta subunit of RNA polymerase (*rpoB*), the latter

of which can also detect common rifampin resistance mutations.[23] IS6110 is an 81-base pair insertion sequence present in multiple copies in many *M. tuberculosis* strains.[24] Although the yield of molecular testing is lower when organisms are not identified histologically, the sensitivity of some assays is high enough to detect rare organisms that may not be present on the examined sections.[22] In these cases, molecular testing must be guided by the overall histologic findings and clinical suspicion.[25] Numerous NTMs are present in the environment and can cause false positives if FFPE samples are contaminated, highlighting the need for caution in interpreting unusual organisms, particularly in immunocompetent individuals.

FUNGAL INFECTIONS

EPIDEMIOLOGY AND LABORATORY DIAGNOSTICS

Fungal infections of the CNS are typically spread hematogenously through dissemination of angioinvasive skin or lung infections.[26] Less commonly, infections may occur through local invasion, such as from the paranasal sinuses into the frontal lobes. A wide variety of organisms can cause disease, some as true pathogens, but most opportunistically in immunocompromised individuals.[27] Clinical manifestations tend to correlate with size of the organisms, such that yeast are associated with meningitis, pseudohyphae with microabscess and focal infarcts, and true hyphae with arterial thrombosis and large strokes. Cultures of CSF and brain tissue are used to isolate most infections for identification and antibiotic susceptibility testing. However, many organisms require weeks to grow, or may not readily exhibit diagnostic features precluding morphologic speciation. Because of the urgent need for treatment, rapid testing options have been developed including India ink for cryptococcal meningitis, and a variety of antigen tests (eg, cryptococcal antigen).[28] Markers of fungal wall components, such as (1,3)-beta-D-glucan, are useful to support a suspected fungal infection and to help rule out species that produce little or no amounts (eg, *Cryptococcus* spp. and Mucorales).[29]

HISTOLOGIC FEATURES

Surgical tissue from fungal infections is frequently collected from large abscesses or space-occupying lesions for diagnosis and treatment of symptoms. Smaller lesions may also be biopsied in the case of microabscesses, focal infarcts, or leptomeningitis, when a radiologic abnormality is identified and other less-invasive testing is non-diagnostic. The type and degree of inflammation vary with patient immune status, and can range from minimal inflammation with rare lymphocytes and histiocytes to large necrotizing granulomas or abscesses. Fungal forms, including yeast, pseudohyphae, and hyphae, can usually be seen on H&E sections, including intraoperative frozen sections, which typically show minimal staining and refractile cell walls (**Fig. 2**A).[30] Further

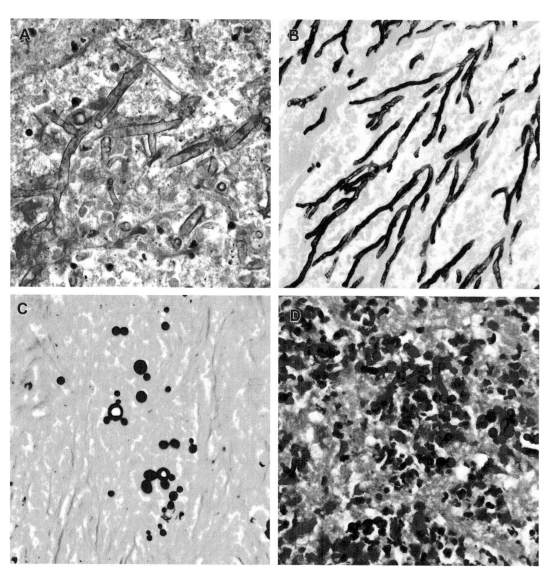

Fig. 2. Fungal infections. (*A*) Fungal forms can often be visualized on standard hematoxylin and eosin stains (original magnification ×400x), as shown in this biopsy of an occipital lobe mass. Wide ribbon-like, pauciseptate hyphae with 90-degree angle branching are present in a necrotic background, consistent with Mucorales infection. Subsequent sequencing of the FFPE tissue targeting the internal transcribed spacer region was positive for *Lichtheimia corymbifera*. (*B*) GMS staining (original magnification ×400x) of tissue from a temporal lobe abscess highlights narrow hyphae with acute-angle branching and frequent septations, consistent with *Aspergillus* spp., further classified as *Aspergillus fumigatus* by culture. (*C*) GMS staining (original magnification ×400x) of a cerebellar abscess biopsy highlights yeast forms with peripheral budding reminiscent of a ship's steering wheel, diagnostic of *Paracoccidioides brasiliensis*. (*D*) Periodic acid–Schiff staining (original magnification ×400x) of a right lobectomy specimen targeting multiple small, radiologically ring-enhancing lesions identified microabscesses containing scattered fungal elements. Medium-to-large, irregular yeast-forms with pseudohypahe are present, suggestive of *Candida* spp. Subsequent sequencing of FFPE using internal transcribed spacer primer sets was positive for *Candida albicans*.

classification is aided by GMS and PAS-D stains, which highlight organism size and morphology (**Fig. 2B–D**). Histologic classification of yeast is based on size and budding pattern (eg, variable-sized yeast with multiple buds of *Paracoccidioides brasiliensis*) (see **Fig. 2**C), and presence of pseudohyphae (eg, *Candida* spp.) (see **Fig. 2**D). Additional staining properties including mucicarmine and Fontana-Masson positivity in *Cryptococcus* spp. and Gram positivity of *Candida* spp. yeast can aid diagnosis, but are not specific and must be interpreted in histologic context.[31] Fungal hyphae are classified by width, branching patterns, frequency of septations, and presence of pigmentation.[32] Mucorales (eg, *Rhizopus* spp. and *Mucor* spp.) exhibit wide, irregular ribbon-like, pauciseptate hyphae with 90-degree angle branching (see **Fig. 2**A). *Aspergillus* spp. exhibit narrow, regular hyphae with frequent septations and 45-degree angle branching (see **Fig. 2**B); however, these features are not specific, and in the absence of supportive laboratory findings, it is recommended to report a morphologic description with a differential including *Fusarium* spp., *Scedosporium* spp., and other hyaline molds. Immunohistochemistry can be performed for fungal identification, but because of substantial cross-reactivity between species offers limited additional information beyond morphologic identification.[33]

MOLECULAR DIAGNOSTICS

Species-level identification of fungi from FFPE is accomplished by sequencing of rRNA genes.[34] Unlike bacterial 16S rRNA sequencing of the small subunit, fungal identification typically relies on the D1/D2 region of the large subunit (28S rRNA gene), and the internal transcribed spacer region, because of increased variation between species. Clinical and Laboratory Standards Institute guidelines have been published for fungal sequencing identification.[14] Additional targets may be necessary to classify beyond complexes, including β-tubulin, calmodulin, or actin for *Aspergillus* spp. In addition to the challenges of sequencing formalin-fixed tissue, fungal cell walls provide an additional barrier and challenge to sequencing, which requires additional steps for adequate lysis and release of fungal nucleic acids.[35] Various physical (eg, beads), chemical/enzymatic, and temperature-based methods have been used to increase yield of fungal DNA extraction. Because even small yeast forms are identified by GMS or PAS-D stains, there is little utility in fungal sequencing of tissue that lacks visible organism. Even in the setting of compatible inflammatory

patterns, molecular testing results are more likely to be false positives because of contamination of reagents or nonsterile collection sites than true infections.[36]

VIRAL INFECTIONS

EPIDEMIOLOGY AND LABORATORY DIAGNOSTICS

Numerous RNA and DNA viruses can infect the CNS of immunocompromised and healthy individuals, manifesting as meningitis, encephalitis, or myelitis.[37] Symptoms are predominantly neurologic or part of a disseminated systemic infection, and can occur either as an acute infection or as a reactivation event because of decreased immune system function. Infections frequently diffusely involve the entire brain via hematogenous spread, but may also exhibit some anatomic predilections, including temporal lobes for herpes simplex virus and thalami/basal ganglia for West Nile virus.[38] Viruses can also exhibit varying levels of tropism for different cell types, such as JC virus in oligodendrocytes, causing white matter–predominant disease as progressive multifocal leukoencephalopathy, and poliovirus infecting anterior horn cells of the spinal cord as poliomyelitis.[39] CSF testing showing a lymphocyte predominance is typical for CNS viral infections, and a specific pathogen may be diagnosed by the presence of CSF antibodies or viral nucleic acids.[40] Detection of IgM in serum or CSF is often the test of choice for viruses with short viremic windows, including most arboviruses; however, immunomodulatory drugs, such as rituximab, an anti-CD20 monoclonal antibody, can decrease the ability to produce antibodies resulting in false-negative testing.[40] Cultures can detect some viruses, but are less sensitive and more time consuming to perform compared with molecular methods, limiting overall utility.[41]

HISTOLOGIC FEATURES

Surgical biopsies are rarely undertaken for the diagnosis of CNS viral infections, because of the high yield of CSF testing with substantially lower costs and morbidity.[42] Biopsy tissue may be obtained to shed light on the cause of a radiologic abnormality for which all less-invasive testing has been unrevealing, and typically encompasses a broad differential, such as glioma, lymphoma, infections, demyelinating, or toxic/metabolic etiologies. In cases with severe edema and risk of death caused by herniation, tissue may be obtained during decompressive surgery. On rare occasions, biopsies of "nonlesional" tissue are obtained, most often from the frontal lobes or other accessible locations, with the goal of identifying a diffuse process, such as vasculitis.[43] General histologic features include varying amounts of perivascular, parenchymal, and leptomeningeal chronic inflammatory infiltrates; microgliosis with microglial nodules and neuronophagia; and neuronal loss (Fig. 3A, B). Inflammatory infiltrates

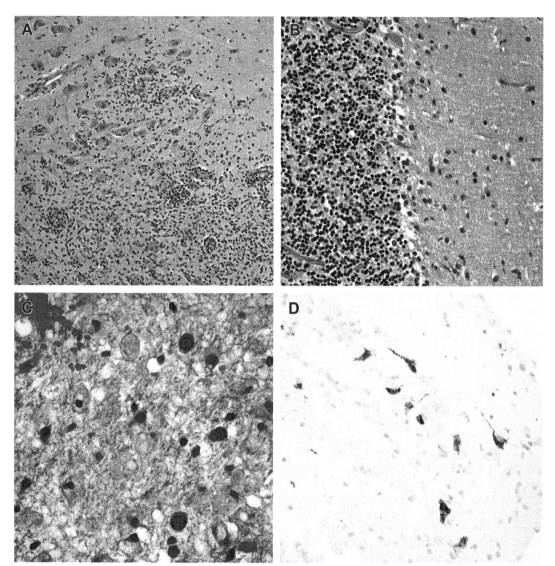

Fig. 3. Viral infections. Many viral infections of the central nervous system show overlapping histologic features with autoimmune encephalitis, precluding further classification without immunohistochemistry or molecular testing. (*A*) This temporal lobe biopsy shows a dense lymphoplasmacytic infiltrate with microglial nodules and neuronophagia of unclear cause (original magnification ×200x). (*B*) Extensive neuronal loss, as in this cerebellar biopsy showing Purkinje cell depletion and Bergmann gliosis, is another nonspecific finding that is seen in viral meningoencephalitis. Metagenomic next-generation sequencing of cerebrospinal fluid and formalin-fixed paraffin-embedded brain tissue was positive for Powassan virus (original magnification ×400x). (*C*) Some viral infections show characteristic viral cytopathic effects that can aid in diagnosis, including JC virus intranuclear inclusions present in oligodendrocytes in this left parietal lesion biopsy. Immunohistochemistry can help distinguish inclusions from reactive nuclei, and confirm specificity for polyomaviruses. Combined with myelin pallor and extensive macrophage infiltration (not shown), these findings are diagnostic of progressive multifocal leukoencephalopathy (original magnification ×400x). (*D*) Herpes simplex virus immunohistochemistry of a temporal lobe biopsy highlights scattered cells containing viral antigen, including neurons, confirming the diagnosis of herpes simplex virus-1 meningoencephalitis (original magnification ×200x).

are generally mixed and include lymphocytes (enriched for CD8[+] T cells), plasma cells, histiocytes, microglia, and may include neutrophils. In severely immunosuppressed individuals, inflammation may be minimal. Demyelination, confirmed by loss of Luxol fast blue staining, is a prominent feature of progressive multifocal leukoencephalopathy, but is also observed in noninfectious (ie, multiple sclerosis) or postinfectious (ie, acute disseminated encephalomyelitis) settings.[44] Vasculitis or ischemic lesions may be present in varicella zoster virus infections.[45] For practical considerations, viruses are often divided into ones that are diagnosed based on histology alone and ones that require ancillary testing in the form of immunohistochemistry or molecular assays. Viral cytopathic effects including nuclear or cytoplasmic inclusions are pathognomonic for certain infections, such as the oligodendrocyte nuclear inclusions of JC virus (**Fig. 3C**), and neuronal cytoplasmic Negri body inclusions of rabies virus. Less specific cytopathic effects, such as multinucleated cells of HIV encephalitis and measles virus, may require confirmation by immunohistochemistry. Similarly, inclusions of herpes simplex virus-1/2, varicella zoster virus, cytomegalovirus, and adenovirus are seen on routine H&E sections, but are easily highlighted by immunohistochemistry (**Fig. 3D**).[46] A large number of other viruses, including human herpesvirus-6/7, enteroviruses, and arboviruses require immunohistochemistry or molecular testing for diagnosis.

MOLECULAR DIAGNOSTICS

Because of the large diversity of virus genomes and lack of common genes across all families, no universal targeted gene sequencing for viruses exists that would be analogous to 16S rRNA for bacteria. Instead, individual or panels of real-time PCR assays have been developed, with or without a sequencing step, for a wide range of viral infections. Specific testing is guided by epidemiologic factors including immune status, age, geography, and exposures. Although these tests are reasonably sensitive and specific, they lack the ability to detect novel viruses, or unusual viruses that were not specifically targeted because of low probability and limited tissue availability. Metagenomic next-generation sequencing (mNGS) has recently become available as a clinical assay for CSF specimens, and has resulted in diagnoses of unexpected pathogens that would otherwise have left the cases unsolved.[47] Sensitivity of mNGS depends on acuity of infection, extent of prior antiviral treatment, and levels of virus shed into the CSF. mNGS assays for fresh/frozen or FFPE brain

tissue are currently being developed, and are likely to have higher yield for ongoing infections and for viruses that exist predominantly intraparenchymaly in the brain.[48] Compared with CSF, brain tissue has a much higher percentage of human to nonhuman nucleic acids, requiring additional purification or bioinformatics steps to identify sequences from potential pathogens.[49] As for other pathogen types, formalin-fixation decreases the length of sequencing reads, although the ability to screen tissue for histologic signs of viral infection may offset this effect. Caution should be used in attributing low levels of human herpesvirus-6 or other viruses that retain latency as causes of acute meningoencephalitis, because these may reflect limited reactivation secondary to other immunosuppressive factors.[50] Although few targeted antiviral therapies are currently available, identification of a specific virus can help limit unnecessary further testing and provide evidence against immunosuppressive treatment of a possible autoimmune encephalitis.

PARASITIC INFECTIONS

EPIDEMIOLOGY AND LABORATORY DIAGNOSTICS

Several parasites can infect the CNS, variably manifesting as benign space-occupying masses to rapidly progressive destructive lesions.[51] Parasites differ widely in geographic distribution, which is heavily influenced by susceptible hosts and vectors, many of which can infect humans as part of a normal or aberrant life cycle. Basic organizational schemes split parasites into single-celled protozoans, including *Toxoplasma* spp., *Plasmodium* spp., and free-living amebas, and macroscopic helminths, which include nematodes (roundworms), cestodes (tapeworms), and trematodes (flukes). As with other types of infections, immunosuppression is associated with more severe infections and infections with unusual organisms.[52] Toxoplasmosis commonly involves the brain in HIV-positive individuals and can present as ring-enhancing lesions on MRI.[53] *Plasmodium falciparum* causes cerebral malaria, particularly in children, because of sequestration in CNS blood vessels.[54] Cysticerci, larval stage of pork tapeworm *Taeni solium*, can present as single or numerous cystic lesions on imaging, and are a major source of seizures worldwide.[55] Free-living amebas, including *Acanthamoeba* spp., *Balamuthia mandrillaris*, and *Naegleria fowleri*, are associated with exposure to fresh, stagnant water, and present with rapid clinical deterioration.[56] Diagnosis is often accomplished using serology, based on exposures to travel, food, and animals/insects. Serum and CSF may show a marked increase in eosinophils, and organisms may be directly observed on peripheral blood smears or detectable by targeted PCR (eg, *Toxoplasma* spp. and *Plasmodium* spp.). Organisms are diagnosed morphologically in the microbiology/hematology laboratories, although cultures do not play a routine role in diagnosis. Treatments range from innocuous trimethoprim-sulfamethoxazole for

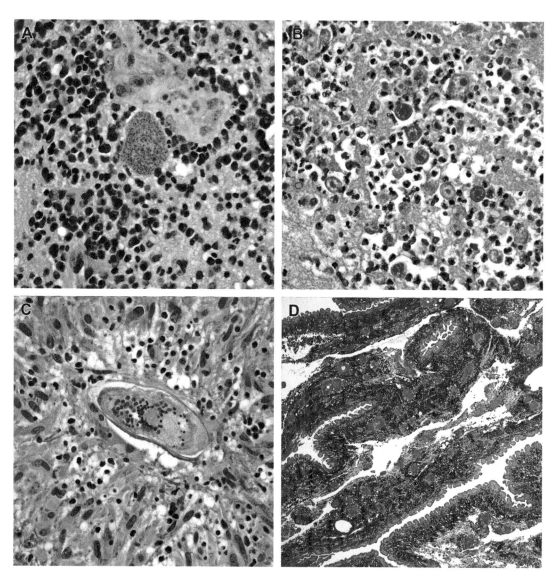

Fig. 4. Parasitic infections. Most parasitic infections of the central nervous system are diagnosed by morphologic features on hematoxylin and eosin sections, with occasional confirmation by serology or molecular testing. (*A*) This biopsy of a temporal lobe mass shows a dense lymphoplasmacytic infiltrate surrounding a thin-walled cyst containing numerous *Toxoplasma gondii* bradyzoites. Immunohistochemistry is used to highlight individual tachyzoites when bradyzoites are not readily identified, and to distinguish from other similarly appearing parasites, such as in trypanosomiasis (original magnification ×400x). (*B*) Autopsy sections from a fatal case of granulomatous amebic encephalitis show numerous trophozoites of *Balamuthia mandrillaris*, which resemble macrophages but contain a large nucleus with distinctive central karyosome (original magnification ×400x). (*C*) Temporal lobe biopsy sections show a marked granulomatous and mixed inflammatory reaction to *Schistosoma mansoni* eggs, which are characterized by oval shape and refractory wall. The location of spines, useful for differentiating among *Schistosoma* spp., are difficult to assess in FFPE sections, which may not contain an optimally oriented egg (original magnification ×400x). (*D*) Tissue from the resection of a large cerebellar cyst shows tegument, stroma, and occasional calcareous bodies without an observable protoscolex, findings consistent with the racemose form of neurocysticercosis (metacestode form of *Taenia solium*) (original magnification ×100x).

toxoplasmosis, to highly toxic and occasionally deadly melarsoprol for trypanosomiasis.[57]

HISTOLOGIC FEATURES

Surgical biopsies or resections may be undertaken for diagnosis and treatment of various radiologic abnormalities. Ring-enhancing lesions encompass a broad infectious and noninfectious differential, including toxoplasmosis.[58] Cystic lesions, such as echinococcosis and cysticercosis, may consist predominantly of fluid and contain extensively degenerated, but distinctly nonhuman appearing tissue. Inflammatory patterns depend on immune status, and range from minimal acute inflammation, to granulomatous inflammation and large areas of necrosis and abscess. Organisms may be found in brain parenchyma, blood vessels, or leptomeninges. Protozoan parasites are frequently recognized on H&E stains; may be intracellular (eg, *Toxoplasma* bradyzoites) (**Fig. 4**A) or extracellular (eg, *Acanthamoeba* spp. trophozoites and cysts) (**Fig. 4**B); and are distinguished based on morphologic features including size, shape, and subcellular organelles. Helminths can be present as eggs (**Fig. 4**C) or larvae/adult worms (**Fig. 4**D), and are distinguished based on size, shape, and presence of various structures including protoscoleces. Special stains, such as Giemsa, may be used to highlight protozoan morphology, acid-fast stains are used to stain the polarizable hooklets present in cestodes, and PAS and GMS stains are used to stain the cyst walls of amebas. Immunohistochemistry for *Toxoplasma* spp. is widely available, and can help highlight tachyzoites in a necrotic background, whereas amebas are distinguished from histiocytes by lack of CD68 staining. Other immunostains may be available at reference laboratories, including assays for specific ameba species.[59] Although no longer a frequent tool for diagnosis, electron microscopy is used to confirm the presence of small, intracellular parasites, such as in microsporidiosis.[60]

MOLECULAR DIAGNOSTICS

Molecular testing is not routinely used for the diagnosis of parasitic infections because of the characteristic histologic features seen in many cases. When only degenerating worm fragments are present precluding further classification (eg, features most consistent with nematode), molecular testing may provide a more specific diagnosis. In such cases, antiparasitic drugs are not indicated unless viable organisms are suspected elsewhere. Some situations for which targeted molecular testing is used include detection of *Toxoplasma gondii* by B1 gene and distinguishing between species of free living amebas by 18S rRNA real-time PCR.[61,62] mNGS has been successful in the diagnosis of parasitic infections from CSF in rare cases, and is likely to be extended to frozen or FFPE brain tissue in the future.[63,64]

SUMMARY

A wide range of organisms can infect the CNS and can cause minimal to lethal symptoms. Although less-invasive testing including CSF examination is preferred whenever possible, surgical biopsy or resection may be used to obtain diagnostic tissue, particularly when neoplastic diagnoses remain in the differential. Histologic evaluation including the use of special stains and immunohistochemistry can identify broad categories of infection (ie, bacterial, mycobacterial, fungal, viral, or parasitic), and can further classify to genus or species in many instances. Targeted molecular testing is used for confirmation in certain settings, whereas broad-spectrum and unbiased metagenomics testing are being increasingly used. Careful histologic review of slides is essential for selecting the ideal molecular test to make a diagnosis and support clinical decision making while minimizing resource overutilization.

ACKNOWLEDGMENTS

No conflicts of interest to declare. No sources of funding supported this work.

DISCLOSURE

The author has nothing to disclose.

REFERENCES

1. Kradin RL. Diagnostic pathology of infectious disease. 2nd edition. Philadelphia: Elsevier; 2018.
2. Procop GW, Pritt BS. Pathology of infectious diseases. Philadelphia: Elsevier/Saunders; 2015.
3. Milner DA, Abedalthagafi M, Pecora N, et al. Diagnostic pathology. infectious diseases. 2nd edition. Philadelphia: Elsevier; 2019.
4. Figueiredo AHA, Brouwer MC, van de Beek D. Acute community-acquired bacterial meningitis. Neurol Clin 2018;36(4):809–20.
5. Brook I. Microbiology and treatment of brain abscess. J Clin Neurosci 2017;38:8–12.
6. Bishop B, Geffen Y, Plaut A, et al. The use of matrix-assisted laser desorption/ionization time-of-flight mass spectrometry for rapid bacterial identification in patients with smear-positive bacterial meningitis. Clin Microbiol Infect 2018;24(2):171–4.

7. Leber AL, Everhart K, Balada-Llasat JM, et al. Multicenter evaluation of biofire filmarray meningitis/encephalitis panel for detection of bacteria, viruses, and yeast in cerebrospinal fluid specimens. J Clin Microbiol 2016;54(9):2251–61.

8. Rath TJ, Hughes M, Arabi M, et al. Imaging of cerebritis, encephalitis, and brain abscess. Neuroimaging Clin N Am 2012;22(4):585–607.

9. Rosa G, Procop GW, Schold JD, et al. Secondary syphilis in HIV positive individuals: correlation with histopathologic findings, CD4 counts, and quantity of treponemes in microscopic sections. J Cutan Pathol 2016;43(10):847–51.

10. Seferovic MD, Pace RM, Carroll M, et al. Visualization of microbes by 16S in situ hybridization in term and preterm placentas without intraamniotic infection. Am J Obstet Gynecol 2019;221(2):146.e1–23.

11. Racsa LD, DeLeon-Carnes M, Hiskey M, et al. Identification of bacterial pathogens from formalin-fixed, paraffin-embedded tissues by using 16S sequencing: retrospective correlation of results to clinicians' responses. Hum Pathol 2017;59:132–8.

12. Do H, Dobrovic A. Sequence artifacts in DNA from formalin-fixed tissues: causes and strategies for minimization. Clin Chem 2015;61(1):64–71.

13. Salipante SJ, Kawashima T, Rosenthal C, et al. Performance comparison of Illumina and ion torrent next-generation sequencing platforms for 16S rRNA-based bacterial community profiling. Appl Environ Microbiol 2014;80(24):7583–91.

14. CLSI. Interpretative criteria for identification of bacteria and fungi by targeted DNA sequencing. CLSI guideline MM18. 2nd edition. Wayne (PA): Clinical and Laboratory Standards Institute; 2018.

15. Drengenes C, Wiker HG, Kalananthan T, et al. Laboratory contamination in airway microbiome studies. BMC Microbiol 2019;19(1):187.

16. Leonard J. Central nervous system tuberculosis. Microbiol Spectr 2017;5(2). https://doi.org/10.1128/microbiolspec.TNMI7-0044-2017.

17. Sheron MW, Holt SL, Ingram CW. Mycobacterium bovis cerebellar abscess following treatment with bacillus Calmette-Guerin. J Pharm Pract 2017; 30(3):378–80.

18. Polavarapu K, Preethish-Kumar V, Vengalil S, et al. Brain and spinal cord lesions in leprosy: a magnetic resonance imaging-based study. Am J Trop Med Hyg 2019;100(4):921–31.

19. Procop GW. Laboratory diagnosis and susceptibility testing for Mycobacterium tuberculosis. Microbiol Spectr 2016;4(6). https://doi.org/10.1128/microbiolspec.TNMI7-0022-2016.

20. Griffith DE, Aksamit T, Brown-Elliott BA, et al. An official ATS/IDSA statement: diagnosis, treatment, and prevention of nontuberculous mycobacterial diseases. Am J Respir Crit Care Med 2007;175(4):367–416.

21. Horne DJ, Kohli M, Zifodya JS, et al. Xpert MTB/RIF and Xpert MTB/RIF Ultra for pulmonary tuberculosis and rifampicin resistance in adults. Cochrane Database Syst Rev 2019;(6). CD009593.

22. Solomon IH, Johncilla ME, Hornick JL, et al. The utility of immunohistochemistry in mycobacterial infection: a proposal for multimodality testing. Am J Surg Pathol 2017;41(10):1364–70.

23. Slany M, Pavlik I. Molecular detection of nontuberculous mycobacteria: advantages and limits of a broad-range sequencing approach. J Mol Microbiol Biotechnol 2012;22(4):268–76.

24. Thierry D, Brisson-Noel A, Vincent-Levy-Frebault V, et al. Characterization of a Mycobacterium tuberculosis insertion sequence, IS6110, and its application in diagnosis. J Clin Microbiol 1990;28(12):2668–73.

25. Miller K, Harrington SM, Procop GW. Acid-fast smear and histopathology results provide guidance for the appropriate use of broad-range polymerase chain reaction and sequencing for mycobacteria. Arch Pathol Lab Med 2015;139(8):1020–3.

26. Raman Sharma R. Fungal infections of the nervous system: current perspective and controversies in management. Int J Surg 2010;8(8):591–601.

27. Chakrabarti A. Epidemiology of central nervous system mycoses. Neurol India 2007;55(3):191–7.

28. Rajasingham R, Wake RM, Beyene T, et al. Cryptococcal meningitis diagnostics and screening in the era of point-of-care laboratory testing. J Clin Microbiol 2019;57(1), [pii:e01238-18].

29. Lyons JL, Thakur KT, Lee R, et al. Utility of measuring (1,3)-beta-d-glucan in cerebrospinal fluid for diagnosis of fungal central nervous system infection. J Clin Microbiol 2015;53(1):319–22.

30. Guarner J, Brandt ME. Histopathologic diagnosis of fungal infections in the 21st century. Clin Microbiol Rev 2011;24(2):247–80.

31. Bishop JA, Nelson AM, Merz WG, et al. Evaluation of the detection of melanin by the Fontana-Masson silver stain in tissue with a wide range of organisms including Cryptococcus. Hum Pathol 2012;43(6):898–903.

32. Chavez JA, Brat DJ, Hunter SB, et al. Practical diagnostic approach to the presence of hyphae in neuropathology specimens with three illustrative cases. Am J Clin Pathol 2018;149(2):98–104.

33. Schuetz AN, Cohen C. Aspergillus immunohistochemistry of culture-proven fungal tissue isolates shows high cross-reactivity. Appl Immunohistochem Mol Morphol 2009;17(6):524–9.

34. Wickes BL, Wiederhold NP. Molecular diagnostics in medical mycology. Nat Commun 2018;9(1):5135.

35. Munoz-Cadavid C, Rudd S, Zaki SR, et al. Improving molecular detection of fungal DNA in formalin-fixed paraffin-embedded tissues: comparison of five tissue DNA extraction methods using panfungal PCR. J Clin Microbiol 2010;48(6):2147–53.

36. Czurda S, Smelik S, Preuner-Stix S, et al. Occurrence of fungal DNA contamination in PCR reagents: approaches to control and decontamination. J Clin Microbiol 2016;54(1):148–52.

37. Tyler KL. Acute viral encephalitis. N Engl J Med 2018;379(6):557–66.

38. Lyons JL. Viral meningitis and encephalitis. Continuum (Minneap Minn) 2018;24(5, Neuroinfectious Disease):1284–97.

39. Wollebo HS, White MK, Gordon J, et al. Persistence and pathogenesis of the neurotropic polyomavirus JC. Ann Neurol 2015;77(4):560–70.

40. Kanjilal S, Cho TA, Piantadosi A. Diagnostic testing in central nervous system infection. Semin Neurol 2019;39(3):297–311.

41. Hodinka RL. Point: is the era of viral culture over in the clinical microbiology laboratory? J Clin Microbiol 2013;51(1):2–4.

42. Heth JA. Neurosurgical aspects of central nervous system infections. Neuroimaging Clin N Am 2012;22(4):791–9.

43. Elbers J, Halliday W, Hawkins C, et al. Brain biopsy in children with primary small-vessel central nervous system vasculitis. Ann Neurol 2010;68(5):602–10.

44. Sarbu N, Shih RY, Jones RV, et al. White matter diseases with radiologic-pathologic correlation. Radiographics 2016;36(5):1426–47.

45. Kennedy PGE, Gershon AA. Clinical features of varicella-zoster virus infection. Viruses 2018;10(11), [pii:E609].

46. Solomon IH, Hornick JL, Laga AC. Immunohistochemistry is rarely justified for the diagnosis of viral infections. Am J Clin Pathol 2017;147(1):96–104.

47. Miller S, Naccache SN, Samayoa E, et al. Laboratory validation of a clinical metagenomic sequencing assay for pathogen detection in cerebrospinal fluid. Genome Res 2019;29(5):831–42.

48. Salzberg SL, Breitwieser FP, Kumar A, et al. Next-generation sequencing in neuropathologic diagnosis of infections of the nervous system. Neurol Neuroimmunol Neuroinflamm 2016;3(4):e251.

49. Bodewes R, van Run PR, Schurch AC, et al. Virus characterization and discovery in formalin-fixed paraffin-embedded tissues. J Virol Methods 2015;214:54–9.

50. Agut H, Bonnafous P, Gautheret-Dejean A. Laboratory and clinical aspects of human herpesvirus 6 infections. Clin Microbiol Rev 2015;28(2):313–35.

51. Carpio A, Romo ML, Parkhouse RM, et al. Parasitic diseases of the central nervous system: lessons for clinicians and policy makers. Expert Rev Neurother 2016;16(4):401–14.

52. Muehlenbachs A, Bhatnagar J, Agudelo CA, et al. Malignant transformation of *Hymenolepis nana* in a human host. N Engl J Med 2015;373(19):1845–52.

53. Bowen LN, Smith B, Reich D, et al. HIV-associated opportunistic CNS infections: pathophysiology, diagnosis and treatment. Nat Rev Neurol 2016;12(11):662–74.

54. Bruneel F. Human cerebral malaria: 2019 mini review. Rev Neurol (Paris) 2019;175(7–8):445–50.

55. Garcia HH, O'Neal SE, Noh J, et al, Cysticercosis Working Group in Peru. Laboratory diagnosis of neurocysticercosis (*Taenia solium*). J Clin Microbiol 2018;56(9), [pii:e00424-18].

56. Trabelsi H, Dendana F, Sellami A, et al. Pathogenic free-living amoebae: epidemiology and clinical review. Pathol Biol (Paris) 2012;60(6):399–405.

57. Babokhov P, Sanyaolu AO, Oyibo WA, et al. A current analysis of chemotherapy strategies for the treatment of human African trypanosomiasis. Pathog Glob Health 2013;107(5):242–52.

58. Khosrodad N, Khine J, Maclean J, et al. When do ring-enhancing brain lesions need to be biopsied, and should they be treated empirically first? Eur J Case Rep Intern Med 2019;6(4):001068.

59. Guarner J, Bartlett J, Shieh WJ, et al. Histopathologic spectrum and immunohistochemical diagnosis of amebic meningoencephalitis. Mod Pathol 2007;20(12):1230–7.

60. Weber R, Deplazes P, Flepp M, et al. Cerebral microsporidiosis due to *Encephalitozoon cuniculi* in a patient with human immunodeficiency virus infection. N Engl J Med 1997;336(7):474–8.

61. Norgan AP, Sloan LM, Pritt BS. Detection of *Naegleria fowleri*, *Acanthamoeba* spp, and *Balamuthia mandrillaris* in formalin-fixed, paraffin-embedded tissues by real-time multiplex polymerase chain reaction. Am J Clin Pathol 2019;152(6):799–807.

62. Liu Q, Wang ZD, Huang SY, et al. Diagnosis of toxoplasmosis and typing of *Toxoplasma gondii*. Parasit Vectors 2015;8:292.

63. Wilson MR, Shanbhag NM, Reid MJ, et al. Diagnosing *Balamuthia mandrillaris* encephalitis with metagenomic deep sequencing. Ann Neurol 2015;78(5):722–30.

64. Wilson MR, O'Donovan BD, Gelfand JM, et al. Chronic meningitis investigated via metagenomic next-generation sequencing. JAMA Neurol 2018;75(8):947–55.

Molecular Advances in Central Nervous System Mesenchymal Tumors

Jeffrey Helgager, MD, PhD[a], Joseph Driver, MD[b],
Samantha Hoffman, BS[b], Wenya Linda Bi, MD, PhD[b],*

KEYWORDS

• Meningioma • Solitary fibrous tumor • Hemangioblastoma • Genomics

Key points

- Integrated molecular, genomic, and immunologic models of meningioma complement classic histopathologic grading schemas in predicting prognosis.

- Benign meningiomas are characterized by recurrent putative oncogenic mutations while aggressive meningiomas feature recurrent chromosomal gains and losses as well as distinct epigenetic signatures, suggestive of distinct pathways for tumorigenesis.

- The NAB2-STAT6 gene fusion is pathognomonic of solitary fibrous tumors, although the molecular drivers of aggressive variants of these tumors remain to be elucidated.

ABSTRACT

Mesenchymal tumors of the central nervous system (CNS) comprise an array of neoplasms that may arise from or secondarily affect the CNS and its immediate surroundings. This review focuses on meningiomas and solitary fibrous tumors, the most common primary CNS mesenchymal tumors, and discusses recent advances in unveiling the molecular landscapes of these neoplasms. An effort is made to underscore those molecular findings most relevant to tumor diagnostics and prognostication from a practical perspective. As molecular techniques become more readily used at the clinical level, such alterations may strengthen formal grading schemes and lend themselves to treatment with targeted therapies.

Mesenchymal tumors are composed of diverse neoplasms that may arise anywhere throughout the body. Some originate from or secondarily affect the central nervous system

(CNS) and its immediate surroundings, including dura, bone, and soft tissue. The most commonly encountered primary mesenchymal tumors of CNS origin are meningioma, the most common primary brain tumor in adults within the United States,[1] followed by solitary fibrous tumors (SFTs), which account for fewer than 1% of intracranial neoplasms.[2] Recent discoveries have shed greater insight into the molecular landscapes underlying these 2 tumors. As an exhaustive review of all mesenchymal tumors that may involve the CNS would not be possible in a limited review article, this review focuses on advances in these 2 entities, with an emphasis on underscoring those findings most relevant to tumor diagnostics and prognostication from a practical perspective.

MENINGIOMAS

Meningiomas are the most common primary CNS tumor in adults, occurring at an incidence of approximately 2.3 to 5.5 cases per 100,000 people

[a] Department of Pathology, Brigham and Women's Hospital, Harvard Medical School, Boston, MA, USA;
[b] Center for Skull Base and Pituitary Surgery, Department of Neurosurgery, Brigham and Women's Hospital, Harvard Medical School, Boston, MA, USA
* Corresponding author. Department of Neurosurgery, Brigham and Women's Hospital, 75 Francis Street, Boston, MA 02115.
E-mail address: wbi@bwh.harvard.edu

Surgical Pathology 13 (2020) 291–303
https://doi.org/10.1016/j.path.2020.02.002
1875-9181/20/© 2020 Elsevier Inc. All rights reserved.

surgpath.theclinics.com

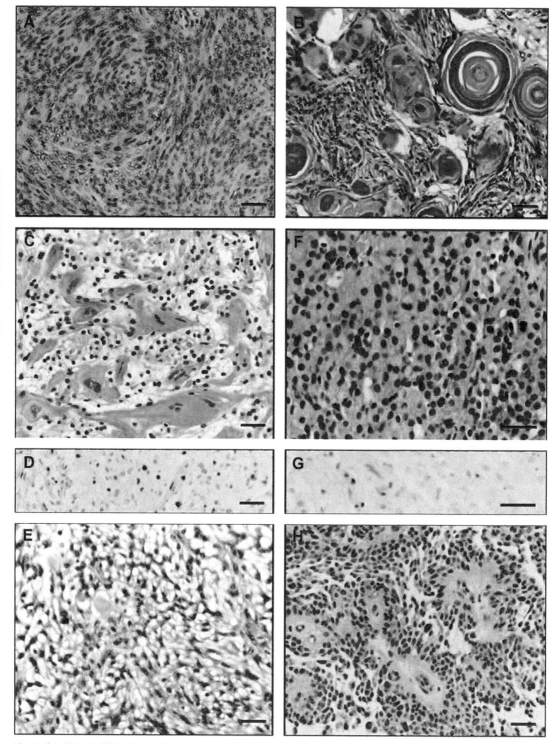

Fig. 1. (*A, B*) Typical histology of meningioma demonstrating whorled and lobulated architecture with a syncytial appearance (meningothelial variant, *A*), sometimes with psammoma bodies (psammomatous variant, *B*). (*C–E*) Grade II histologic variants of meningioma including clear cell meningioma (*C*), in which immunohistochemistry for SMARCE1 frequently demonstrates protein loss in tumor cells (*D*, note preservation of staining in admixed non-neoplastic cells), and chordoid meningioma (*E*). Clear cell meningioma is characterized by clear, glycogen-rich cytoplasm and prominent collagen bundles, whereas chordoid meningioma resembles chordoma and is characterized by trabeculae of vacuolated cells with a mucoid matrix. (*F–H*) Grade III histologic variants of meningioma including rhabdoid meningioma (*F*), in which immunohistochemistry for BAP1 may demonstrate protein loss in tumor cells (*G*, note preservation of staining in admixed non-neoplastic cells), and papillary meningioma (*H*). Rhabdoid meningiomas are characterized by an epithelioid or rhabdoid cytology with prominent nucleoli, whereas papillary meningiomas have a perivascular, pseudopapillary architecture. Other atypical or anaplastic features in these tumors are common. Scale bars = 20 μm.

during their life span.[3,4] Histologically, they are quintessentially characterized by a lobular, whorled architecture with a syncytial appearance, sometimes with psammoma bodies (**Fig. 1**A, B), although numerous variations exist. Although approximately 85% of tumors are World Health Organization (WHO) grade I, and often curable with surgical resection, a portion of these tumors present management challenges.[5] More aggressive meningiomas, classified as WHO grade II-III, exhibit invasive behavior and are prone to recurrence. For those aggressive tumors that recur despite multiple surgeries and radiation therapy, a need for effective adjuvant therapy remains.

Over the past decade, understanding of the molecular drivers of meningioma growth and behavior has grown. Numerous driver mutations have been identified, and modern genetic analysis has demonstrated the presence of a high degree of copy number variations (CNVs), especially in high-grade meningioma. Early studies have suggested that high-grade tumors may exist in an immune-suppressed tumor microenvironment, thereby heralding interest in the application of immunotherapies to meningioma.

EMBRYOLOGY

Meningiomas arise from a cell population within the cerebral meninges, the 3-layered protective covering that lines the CNS. The meninges that cover the cerebral hemispheres are derived from neural crest cells, which are a pluripotent population of cells that delaminate from the neural plate-ectoderm junction to migrate and differentiate into a number of cell types. In contrast, the meninges that line the midbrain and hindbrain are derived from cephalic mesoderm.[6] Classically, meningiomas are believed to originate from the cap cells of the arachnoid layer of the meninges. These cells line the arachnoid villi and protrude into venous sinuses, with the physiologic function of draining cerebrospinal fluid into venous space.

Experimental investigation has identified a common prostaglandin D2 synthase positive (PGDS+) primordial meningeal cell that gives rise to the inner layer of the dura mater (dural border cells) and the outer layer of the arachnoid. These cells are of neural crest origin in the telencephalon and of mesodermal origin in the midbrain. Of note, inactivation of NF2 alone in these PGDS+ precursor cells is sufficient for development of meningothelial and fibroblastic meningiomas in a murine model, supporting their role as a progenitor of meningiomas, and the concept that loss of NF2 is an early driver event in tumorigenesis.[7]

CURRENT HISTOLOGIC GRADING CRITERIA AND LIMITATIONS

Traditionally, the most critical pathologic determination that must be made by the neuropathologist when assessing meningiomas is assignment of grade, an objective means of predicting overall aggressiveness, including likelihood of tumor recurrence. Meningiomas are classically assigned to 1 of 3 grades (WHO grade I–III) based on histologic features, which roughly predict prognostic outcomes: benign meningiomas (grade I) have a 10-year overall survival of approximately 80% to 90%,[8–10] atypical meningiomas (grade II) 53% to 79%,[11–13] and anaplastic meningiomas (grade III) 14% to 34%[11,14]; corresponding progression-

---

Box 1
Meningioma grading criteria

Grade 1 (Benign):

   Mitoses less than 4/10 high-powered fields (HPF)

   AND no other criteria (below) for higher grade fulfilled

Grade II (Atypical):

   Mitoses more than 4/10 HPF but fewer than 20/10 HPF

   OR 3 or more of the following histologic criteria:

   • Increased cellularity

   • Sheetlike growth

   • Prominent nucleoli

   • Small cell change

   • Spontaneous necrosis

   OR one of the following histologic variants:

   • Clear cell meningioma

   • Chordoid meningioma

   OR brain invasion

Grade III (Anaplastic):

   Mitoses more than 20/10 HPF

   OR one of the following histologic variants:

   • Rhabdoid meningioma

   • Papillary meningioma

Adapted from Louis, D.N., et al., *WHO classification of tumours of the central nervous system.* Revised 4th edition. ed. World Health Organization classification of tumours. 2016, Lyon: International Agency For Research On Cancer; with permission.

free survival is 79% to 90% for benign,[8–10] 23% to 78% for atypical,[11–13] and 0% for anaplastic meningiomas.[11,14] Not surprisingly, these outcomes are further influenced by nonhistologic parameters, such as extent of resection, tumor location, age, and use of adjuvant therapies.

The histologic parameters determining meningioma grade have remained almost constant for more than 15 years, with minor nuances (Box 1).[2,15,16] In the most recent, 2016, edition of the *WHO Classification of Tumors of the Central Nervous System*, brain invasion is now deemed sufficient criterion for grade II designation, even in the absence of other atypical features.[2] Previously, such invasion has been associated with adverse prognostic outcome but was not included in formal grading criteria.[15–17]

In practice, the most objective and therefore reliable grading feature is mitotic activity, which is the only parameter that can establish a grade III (anaplastic) diagnosis. Atypical features such as small cell change and sheetlike growth can formally be used to establish a grade II diagnosis when 3 or more are present; however, these are somewhat subjective and caution should be exercised when using them as sole criteria for assigning higher grade; preferably, such features should support a higher grade already determined by mitotic index or presence of brain invasion. In addition, mitotic activity is ideally commensurate with the MIB-1 proliferative index, although their relationship may be inconsistent.

Numerous histologic variants of meningioma are also recognized, with the majority thought to be prognostically inconsequential (see Fig. 1). Those of prognostic importance for the pathologist to report include clear cell and chordoid meningioma, which are grade II tumors by default, as well as rhabdoid and papillary meningioma, which are grade III.[2] Such histologic variants can be diagnosed even in the absence of other atypical or anaplastic features; if the histology is not well-developed or sparsely distributed, the prognostic implications of assigning a higher grade must be weighed. This is exemplified in a study of meningiomas with rhabdoid histology lacking other features of anaplasia, demonstrating that only a subset may be more aggressive than their non-rhabdoid counterparts.[18]

The ambiguity of assigning tumor grade based solely on atypical or aggressive histologic features, and the observation of grade I meningioma recurrence despite benign histopathology and aggressive treatment,[19] highlights the imperfections of the existing morphology-based grading scheme. To counter these limitations, integrated molecular models including genetic mutations, CNV, and methylation profiles have been presented to better predict tumor recurrence.[20–23] We therefore review molecular alterations that inform meningioma grade, aggressiveness, and prognosis (Table 1).

MOLECULAR ALTERATIONS INFORMING MENINGIOMA AGGRESSIVENESS

Cytogenetics

Meningiomas harbor stereotypical chromosomal losses and gains, or CNVs, which inform clinical aggressiveness. Generally, the number of CNVs correlates with histologic grade and risk of tumor recurrence. Grade I tumors have 0 or 1 CNVs, typically monosomy of chromosome 22, whereas grade II and III tumors express an increasing burden of chromosomal alterations.[24–28] Mechanistically, CNVs are presumed to cause dysregulation of oncogene or tumor suppressor gene activity.[29]

Table 1
Molecular alterations associated with meningioma and grade correlations

	Grade 1 (Benign)	Grade II (Atypical)	Grade III (Anaplastic)
Cytogenetics	Monosomy 22	Polysomy Iq, 9q, 12q, 15q, 17q, and 20q Loss of *Ip*, 6q, 10, 14q, and 18q	1–2 copy loss of 9p, including 9p21, encompassing CDKN2A/CDKN2B Amplification of 17q23, encompassing PS6K
Mutations	*NF2* *AKT1, SMO, TRAF7, KLF4, POLR2A*	*SMARCE1* (clear cell meningioma) TERT promoter	*BAP1* (rhabdoid meningioma)

Adapted from Louis, D.N., et al., WHO classification of tumours of the central nervous system. Revised 4th edition. ed. World Health Organization classification of tumours. 2016, Lyon: International Agency For Research On Cancer.

Monosomy 22 is the most commonly observed copy number variation, found in 40% to 70% of meningiomas, and frequently the only cytogenetic abnormality present in grade I tumors.[30,31] The angiomatous histologic subtype offers an exception given their molecular signature of multiple polysomies, despite benign or grade I designation.[32] Atypical and anaplastic meningiomas harbor additional losses in 1p, 6q, 9p, 10, 14q, and 18q with gains in 1q, 9q, 12q, 15q, 17q, and 20q.[2,30] Chromosome 1p and 14q loss are the second and third most common genetic alterations after monosomy 22, respectively. Loss of chromosome 1p has been shown to be associated with higher likelihood of recurrence in grade I tumors, and therefore is thought to be a poor prognostic marker independent of histologic grade.[25,33] Loss of both 22q and 1p is a strong predictor of decreased recurrence-free survival.[21] Genetic mutations driving neoplasia on chromosome 1p in sporadic meningiomas have yet to be identified.

Anaplastic meningiomas are particularly associated with loss of chromosome 9p, including the tumor suppressor proteins CDKN2A, CDK4, and ARF located at 9p21. Even among histologically anaplastic meningiomas, CDKN2A deletion and inactivating mutations were associated with poorer outcome.[34,35] Amplification of 17q23 encompassing the *PS6K* oncogene has also been documented in a small subset of anaplastic meningiomas.[36] Although cytogenetic abnormalities predicting more aggressive behavior are not used for formal grading at this time, their presence in histologically benign tumors is important for the pathologist to note, as these tumors should be regarded as potentially behaving more aggressively.

Molecular Signatures of Aggressive Histologic Variants

The identification of histologic subtypes of meningioma that behave more aggressively and are assigned a higher grade, independent of other aggressive histologic features, suggests that there may be underlying molecular correlates to such variants; these signatures may aid in a more definitive diagnosis as well as yield insights into mechanisms of tumorigenesis. These molecular perturbations were frequently identified as germline mutations in cases of familial meningioma, with subsequent appreciation for their presence in sporadic meningiomas.

Patients with mutations in *SMARCE1*, a gene involved in chromatin remodeling, have a propensity to develop spinal and cranial clear cell meningiomas.[37–39] This has been observed in familial hereditary settings as well as sporadic clear cell meningiomas. In chordoid meningiomas, an unbalanced translocation between chromosomes 1 and 3 has been reported but is not yet defined as a consistent signature.[40]

Inactivating mutations in the BAP1 protein, a tumor suppressor that is a ubiquitin carboxy-terminal hydrolase, have been identified in families with a propensity to develop rhabdoid meningiomas as well as in sporadic rhabdoid meningiomas.[41–43] *BAP1* germline mutations also predispose to uveal and cutaneous melanoma, mesothelioma, and other tumors. Tumors with such inactivating mutations usually also have loss of heterozygosity of chromosome 3p encompassing the *BAP1* gene, and almost uniformly have loss of BAP1 protein expression detectable by immunohistochemistry (IHC). Notably, patients with meningiomas with BAP1 loss were found to have significantly shorter times to progression than those with similar histologic grade with intact BAP1 expression.[41] Furthermore, given there is also some histologic overlap of these tumors with papillary meningiomas,[44] this raises the question if *BAP1* mutations may also be an underlying molecular driver in this subtype. Immunohistochemistry allows ready detection of BAP1 protein loss and may guide identification of more aggressive rhabdoid meningiomas in clinical practice. Patients with BAP1-inactivated rhabdoid meningiomas should be assessed for germline mutations as part of an inherited syndrome.

Genetic Mutations

Beyond cytogenetic alterations and gene mutations associated with more aggressive histologic subtypes, several genetic aberrations have been identified that may predict more aggressive behavior. One such event is activating mutations in the *TERT* promoter, which have been shown to be associated with higher-grade meningiomas, although occur in only a subset of these malignancies.[45–47] Such mutations have been identified in approximately 6.5% to 11.0% of meningiomas, but may reach closer to 20% in grade III tumors.[46,47] TERT encodes telomerase, key to maintaining telomere length, and is a key oncogenic driver in many tumors. Furthermore, regardless of grade, meningiomas with such mutations have been shown to have significantly shorter progression-free survival, and therefore appear to be predictive of poor prognosis.

Alterations of the Switch/sucrose nonfermentable (SWI/SNF) chromatin remodeling complex, which is a family of proteins involved in chromatin remodeling, are observed at higher rates in anaplastic meningiomas, and are associated with worse overall prognosis.[23] Mutations in several members of this complex have been identified, including *SMARCE1*, *SMARCB1*, *SMARCA4*, *PBRM1*, and *ARID1A*.[23,48,49] *SMARCE1*, as discussed previously, is pathognomonic of clear cell meningiomas. In addition, high-grade meningiomas have been found to have upregulation of the polycomb repressive complex 2 (PRC2) and its catalytic domain, which functions in balance with the SWI/SNF complex.[49] The upregulation of PRC2 and downregulation of SWI/SNF demonstrates the important role of chromatin regulation in meningiomas.

Although few other mutations with poor prognostic significance have been recognized, several recurrent genetic mutations have been identified that are associated with meningiomas as a whole and may inform mechanisms of tumorigenesis. Along these lines, no discussion of gene mutations in meningiomas would be complete without mention of *NF2*, the gene encoding the protein Merlin, in which germline inactivating mutations are causal of the syndrome neurofibromatosis type 2. Patients with this syndrome have a predisposition to developing multiple meningiomas,[28] among other neoplasms, which generally have loss of Merlin protein expression through a classic 2-hit event such as acquisition of monosomy 22.[31,50] Interestingly, *NF2* inactivating mutations are also the most common genetic mutations in sporadic meningiomas, occurring in approximately 60% of tumors, and also frequently occur in tandem with loss of heterozygosity of this genetic locus.[51,52] *NF2*-mutant meningiomas are associated with fibrous or transitional histology.[53,54] These mutations appear to be early and likely initiating events in tumorigenesis, and are found roughly equally across all meningioma grades.[55] Notably, numerous other genetically inherited syndromes have also been associated with development of meningiomas, suggesting a multifactorial means of tumorigenesis.

In sporadic meningiomas, other somatic mutations have been identified, including mutations in AKT serine/threonine kinase 1 (*AKT1*), smoothened (*SMO*), tumor necrosis factor (TNF)-receptor associated factor 7 (*TRAF7*), and Kruppel-like factor 4 (*KLF4*).[26,56–58] These tumors comprise approximately 40% of meningiomas, preferentially occur at the skull base, are generally grade I in nature, and are mutually exclusive of *NF2* mutations. Those meningiomas with *AKT1* or *SMO* mutations are enriched along the midline anterior skull base and are frequently meningothelial in histologic subtype. Those with *TRAF7* mutations may have concomitant mutations in *AKT1* or *KLF4*, and

those with the latter are generally of the secretory histologic subtype.[59] Finally, in non-NF2 mutant tumors lacking any of these drivers, recurrent mutations have also been found in *POLR2A*, encoding the catalytic subunit of RNA polymerase II, preferentially associated with sellar tumors and of the meningothelial histologic subtype.[60] Notably, as all of these mutations are found in association with lower grade tumors, their presence may suggest a more benign clinical course.

Last, mutations in *PIK3CA*, a known oncogene mutated in 15% of human cancers[61] has been demonstrated in 4% to 7% of meningiomas,[62,63] leading to constitutive activation of downstream AKT1 and mammalian target of rapamycin (mTOR) signaling and, thus, cellular proliferation and progression through the cell cycle. *PIK3CA* activating mutations appear mutually exclusive of *NF2*, *SMO*, and *AKT1*.[62,63] The *SUFU* gene, which is involved in the hedgehog signaling pathway, has also been found to be mutated in approximately 1% of sporadic meningiomas, with germline mutations present in familial cases.[60]

DNA Methylation

Epigenetic regulation of the genome plays a significant role in gene regulation and cancer biology. Hypermethylation of certain segments of the genome leads to repression of gene expression in those regions, and this has important consequences for tumorigenesis. Global DNA hypomethylation and focal DNA hypermethylation are associated with tumor development, and this has been found in meningioma.[64] Differential methylation status between low-grade and high-grade meningiomas has been identified in important genes including *TMP3*, *CDKN2A*, and *TP73*.[65] Several studies have conducted large-scale methylation profiling and identified separate subclasses of meningiomas following unsupervised clustering analysis. Methylation-based subgroups successfully categorized patients in similar risk groups, and effectively predicted risk for tumor recurrence.[20,66] These findings show that epigenetic characteristics can be an important source of prognostic information. There is great interest in development of a clinically validated methylome-based predictor to aid in clinical decision making; however, such techniques are available at only a handful of institutions at present, and largely remain a research tool.

MOLECULAR MARKERS IN MENINGIOMA DIAGNOSTICS

Although the histologic diagnosis of meningioma is generally straightforward, there can be histologic mimics, the most common of which is solitary fibrous tumor (see later in this article), which occasionally may be confused with the fibrous histologic subtype of meningioma. Therefore, immunohistochemical markers that are sensitive and specific for meningiomas can be of diagnostic value. Meningiomas traditionally stain for epithelial membrane antigen (EMA) and somatostatin receptor 2a (SSTR2a), although degree of staining can be quite variable between individual tumors and higher-grade neoplasms may lose expression; these 2 markers are relatively sensitive and specific in the context of a dural-based mass, although there can be confounders.[67,68] Notably, SFTs should be consistently negative for both EMA and SSTR2a. Another molecular marker for meningiomas readily detectable by IHC is progesterone receptor, expressed in most tumors.[69]

Recently, one study has made inroads toward finding lineage-specific transcription factors expressed in meningiomas, which could also be detected by IHC and aid in the diagnosis of such neoplasms.[70] Such lineage-specific transcription factors are used routinely to identify other neoplasms, such as TTF-1 for lung and thyroid tumors, OLIG-2 for gliomas, and GATA-3 for breast and urothelial cancer. Identified markers include SIX1, FOXC1, MEOX2, which are readily assayable by IHC and therefore could be used in clinical practice. This study demonstrated relative sensitivity and specificity of these markers for meningioma; however, further validation over multiple trials will be necessary.

A COMBINED IMMUNOLOGIC AND GENOMIC APPROACH TO INVESTIGATING MENINGIOMAS

As molecular biology techniques advance in parallel with the rapid progression of genomic analysis, increasing interest has emerged in combining the two approaches to investigate the role of the immune system in mesenchymal tumors. The characterization of the immune *gestalt* of meningiomas date back to the 1980s,[71] but pose several limitations. First, only a handful of studies to date have examined the tumor microenvironment of meningiomas, with limited sample sizes, which hinder the ability to extrapolate these data to all meningiomas. Furthermore, the techniques used in previous investigations, most commonly IHC and flow cytometry, select for limited immunologic markers without ability to explore all possible cell types. Newer protocols that aim to improve this coverage include bulk and single-cell RNA-sequencing, multiplexed immunofluorescence for in situ visualization of immune infiltrates, and

mass cytometry by time of flight for multiple epitope analysis compared with traditional cytometry.

Existing data suggest that the immunophenotype of meningiomas comprise a predominant macrophagic infiltrate.[71–77] Although some investigations indicate a correlation between macrophage density and WHO grade,[71,76,78] others found no such association.[72,75] The antitumoral versus anti-inflammatory, and perhaps protumoral, functionality of the existent macrophage populations in meningioma also merits closer inspection. Similarly, the observed degree of lymphocytic infiltrate and its subpopulations (B cell vs T cell, CD4+ vs CD8+ T-cell predominance) varies significantly between the different studies.[75,79,80]

One possibility for immune variations in meningiomas may derive from the individual genomic makeup of these tumors (**Fig. 2**). For example, PIK3C/AKT pathway signaling contributes to T lymphocyte fate determination: constitutive AKT signaling suppresses the regulatory T-cell lineage in vitro, whereas pharmaceutical inhibition of mTOR promotes effector memory CD8+ T-cell generation as observed in vivo. Given that *AKT1* mutations are largely confined to grade I meningiomas, the possibility arises that the same mutation is at once the tumorigenic driver and an enabler of antitumoral immune responses that inhibit a transition to malignancy. Contradictory to this hypothesis is the finding that the immune checkpoint proteins PD-L2 and B7-H3, which enable tumoral evasion of the immune system, are upregulated in meningiomas with PIK3C/AKT pathway mutations.[81] Further investigation is therefore warranted to understand the immunogenomic dynamics surrounding this signaling cascade.

Similarly, TRAF7 lies downstream of the TNF-alpha cascade and therefore mediates a proinflammatory response (see **Fig. 2**). Constitutive activation of TRAF7 could potentially facilitate a paradoxic oncogenesis and immune attack phenotype as in *AKT1*-mutant tumors. Identification of GREM2 downregulation in higher-grade meningiomas supports the converse of this hypothesis: loss of immune signaling facilitates tumor progression.[82] GREM2 inhibits bone morphogenetic protein (BMP) signaling, which lies upstream of transforming growth factor beta-1 (TGF-β1) expression; this pathway in turn regulates lymphocyte survival and proliferation. Previous studies have established the protective effects of BMP and TGF-β1 activity against meningioma progression; loss of this activity via downregulation of GREM2 could therefore attenuate immunologic efficacy against these tumors, explaining the resulting malignant phenotypes.[82]

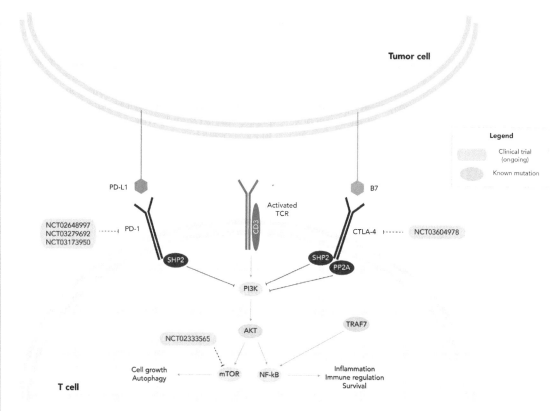

Fig. 2. Immune pathways implicated in meningiomas and current clinical trials targeting those pathways.

The few existing immunogenomic studies of meningiomas support a genomic influence on the immune microenvironment of meningiomas. For instance, a transcriptomic analysis of de novo meningiomas demonstrates enriched expression of genes regulating inflammatory, interferon-gamma, and allograft rejection responses in grade I tumors. Corresponding immunohistochemical staining for CD45, a pan-leukocyte marker, of this cohort supports a differential immune response; grade I tumors had significantly higher infiltration than grade II or III meningiomas.[82] Another group investigating radiation-induced meningiomas carrying NF2-fusion events report significant differences in immunophenotype between their cohorts and meningiomas harboring other known driver mutations. RNA-sequencing analysis indicated increased expression of both inflammatory genes (STAT-4, IGF-1) and immunosuppressive factors (PD-1) in *NF2*-fusion meningiomas,[83] whereas IHC revealed exhaustion of inflammatory cells in the form of increased PD-L1 staining and decreased CD3+ lymphocyte presence compared with non-*NF2*-fusion tumors.[84,85]

Last, tumor transcriptomic analysis and subsequent linear regression revealed immunologic gene expression to be vitally correlated with meningioma location after controlling for WHO grade; specifically, skull base meningiomas displayed significantly higher immune upregulation than did convexity meningiomas.[86] Cytokine-based interrogation of the immune populations at these 2 sites may also reconcile the seemingly contradictory observations of proinflammatory and immunosuppressive myeloid subpopulations from previous data. Antitumoral M1 macrophages were highly correlated to skull base location by network analysis, whereas oncogenic mast cells predominated convexity meningiomas.[86] Together, these data suggest significant variation in immune microenvironment across intracranial sites that may explain historical (albeit controversial) correlations between malignancy and meningioma location.

SOLITARY FIBROUS TUMOR/HEMANGIOPERICYTOMA

SFTs are rare fibroblastic neoplasms most commonly arising within pleura; however, may occur at almost any anatomic site, including the CNS.[87] Those of CNS origin make up less than

1% of primary CNS tumors, and invariably arise from a dural location.[2,88,89] They largely effect middle-aged adults in the fourth and fifth decades of life, with a slight male predominance. Histologically these tumors are monomorphic, spindled cells that take on a jumbled, yet characteristic architecture commonly referred to as a "patternless pattern," separated by thick bands of collagen and thin-walled, staghorn vessels.

The term "hemangiopericytoma" is an obsolete term for these neoplasms when used outside of the CNS, as it historically encompassed a variety of neoplastic entities with similar architectural patterns, including SFTs, all now designated with more specific names[90]; it has been done away with in the realm of soft tissue and pulmonary pathology. Despite this, the term persists in the practice of neuropathology, and up until the 2016 WHO Classification of Tumors of the Central Nervous System, higher-grade SFTs, which were more cellular with less intervening stroma were separately classified as hemangiopericytomas.[16] The finding that almost all of these tumors harbor an NAB2-STAT6 gene fusion, now regarded as a specific and pathognomonic genetic alteration defining SFTs, effectively eliminated hemangiopericytoma as a separate entity. However, only within the CNS, SFTs presently are formally classified as solitary fibrous tumor/hemangiopericytoma in the 2016 WHO classification[2]; this classification will likely be done away with in future editions.

GRADING

Grading of SFTs within the CNS, like formal nomenclature, is also different from those at other anatomic sites. CNS SFTs are graded from WHO grade I-III, with a distinction between those of traditional SFT histology (grade I, benign) or hemangiopericytoma histology (grade II or III, malignant),[2] although admittedly such morphologic phenotypes are not always discrete and there is a phenotypic spectrum. The importance of this distinction rests on studies demonstrating that those of SFT phenotype display benign behavior with little likelihood of recurrence given full surgical resection, whereas those of hemangiopericytoma phenotype have a significant risk of recurrence and metastasis (>70% recurrence with 10-year follow-up with ~20% of patients developing extracranial metastases). Further distinction between grade II and III tumors rests on mitotic count, with more than 5 mitoses/10 high-powered fields (HPF) achieving a grade III designation.

Outside the CNS, a distinction between SFT and hemangiopericytoma histology is not made, with mitotic count (>4/10 HPFs) being the most important prognostic determinant of malignancy.[87,91] The prognostic relevance of mitotic count has also been demonstrated in SFTs of the CNS, independent of other parameters, including histologic phenotype.[92] An argument for aligning grading criteria for CNS SFTs with those used at other anatomic sites could thus be made. Along these lines, whether a recently proposed and widely adopted risk stratification model for nonmeningeal SFTs is relevant to CNS tumors also remains an open question worthy of further study.[93]

MOLECULAR MARKERS OF SOLITARY FIBROUS TUMORS

Until 2013, a molecular signature for SFTs remained elusive, although immunohistochemically they were known typically to express CD34 and CD99 with a subset positive for Bcl-2, none of these markers sensitive or specific for this entity.[90] A major breakthrough in the understanding of the molecular signature of these tumors arose with the identification of a chromosomal inversion at the 12q13 locus in the vast majority of these neoplasms, resulting in fusion of the NAB2 and STAT6 genes.[94–96] Numerous variations of this translocation have been identified, all of which result in the nuclear localization domain of NAB2 being fused to STAT6, a cytoplasmic transcription factor. The result is nuclear localization of the resulting fusion protein and transcriptional activation; this fusion product has been demonstrated to induce proliferation in cell culture and is likely the initiating driver in SFT tumorigenesis.[94] Notably, NAB2 and STAT6 are positioned in close proximity on chromosome 12, and thus molecular tests, such as fluorescence in situ hybridization, may give false negative results. To this end, IHC demonstrating nuclear localization of STAT6 seems to be an even more sensitive and specific surrogate marker for the presence of this fusion transcript, and absence of this marker in a suspected SFT should call such a diagnosis into question.[97,98]

MOLECULAR MARKERS INFORMING SOLITARY FIBROUS TUMOR AGGRESSIVENESS

Given an evolving understanding of histologic determinants of SFT aggressiveness within the CNS, molecular determinants informing malignant potential would be invaluable for grading and prognostication. Compared with meningiomas, aggressive molecular signatures of SFTs are more sparsely understood, in part because of the relative rarity of these tumors. In a study of nonmeningeal SFTs,[99] the most common NAB2-STAT6 fusion, NAB2ex4-STAT6ex2/3, was observed in tumors with classic SFT histology, a less aggressive clinical course, and an older patient population. The NAB2ex6-STAT6ex16/17 fusion, in contrast, was associated with hemangiopericytoma histology, more aggressive behavior, and found in younger patients. Subsequent study of meningeal SFTs found similar correlations, although no prognostic significance was detected, likely due to small sample size.[100] Importantly, such fusion variants target different functional domains of both the NAB2 and STAT6 genes, thereby providing a functional molecular correlate by which variable oncogenicity could be conferred. As in meningiomas, *TERT* promoter mutations have recently been documented in SFTs and appear to confer increased aggressiveness.[101,102] Such alterations might be incorporated into future grading schemes, as molecular methods become more accessible to general pathology practice.

SUMMARY

The past several years have seen numerous developments in the discovery of molecular alterations both defining meningiomas and SFTs, as well as those that may predict tumor aggressiveness. As techniques of molecular biology become more readily used at the clinical level, such alterations undoubtedly will become formally incorporated into tumor grading and prognostication, including even now cutting-edge technologies such as DNA methylation profiling. In addition, as molecular profiling of these tumors becomes more commonplace and more tumors are routinely profiled, further insights into such molecular alterations, how they drive tumorigenesis, and how they may predict aggressiveness as well as susceptibility to targeted therapies will be further gained.

REFERENCES

1. Ostrom QT, Gittleman H, Truitt G, et al. CBTRUS statistical report: primary brain and other central nervous system tumors diagnosed in the United States in 2011-2015. Neuro Oncol 2018; 20(suppl_4):iv1–86.
2. Louis DN, Ohgaki H, Wiestler OD, et al. WHO classification of tumours of the central nervous system. In: World Health Organization classification of tumours. Revised 4th edition. Lyon: International Agency For Research On Cancer; 2016. p. 408.
3. Kurland LT, Schoenberg BS, Annegers JF, et al. The incidence of primary intracranial neoplasms in Rochester, Minnesota, 1935-1977. Ann N Y Acad Sci 1982;381:6–16.
4. Sutherland GR, Florell R, Choi NW, et al. Epidemiology of primary intracranial neoplasms in Manitoba, Canada. Can J Neurol Sci 1987;14(4):586–92.
5. Bi WL, Abedalthagafi M, Horowitz P, et al. Genomic landscape of intracranial meningiomas. J Neurosurg 2016;125(3):525–35.
6. Richtsmeier JT, Flaherty K. Hand in glove: brain and skull in development and dysmorphogenesis. Acta Neuropathol 2013;125(4):469–89.
7. Kalamarides M, Stemmer-Rachamimov AO, Niwa-Kawakita M, et al. Identification of a progenitor cell of origin capable of generating diverse meningioma histological subtypes. Oncogene 2011; 30(20):2333–44.
8. Rogers L, Barani I, Chamberlain M, et al. Meningiomas: knowledge base, treatment outcomes, and uncertainties. A RANO review. J Neurosurg 2015; 122(1):4–23.
9. Tanzler E, Morris CG, Kirwan JM, et al. Outcomes of WHO Grade I meningiomas receiving definitive or postoperative radiotherapy. Int J Radiat Oncol Biol Phys 2011;79(2):508–13.
10. van Alkemade H, de Leau M, Dieleman EMT, et al. Impaired survival and long-term neurological problems in benign meningioma. Neuro Oncol 2012; 14(5):658–66.
11. Durand A, Labrousse F, Jouvet A, et al. WHO grade II and III meningiomas: a study of prognostic factors. J Neurooncol 2009;95(3):367–75.
12. Sun SQ, Cai C, Murphy RKJ, et al. Management of atypical cranial meningiomas, part 2: predictors of progression and the role of adjuvant radiation after subtotal resection. Neurosurgery 2014;75(4):356–63, [discussion: 363].
13. Sun SQ, Kim AH, Cai C, et al. Management of atypical cranial meningiomas, part 1: predictors of recurrence and the role of adjuvant radiation after gross total resection. Neurosurgery 2014;75(4):347–54, [discussion: 354-5; quiz: 355].
14. Palma L, Celli P, Franco C, et al. Long-term prognosis for atypical and malignant meningiomas: a study of 71 surgical cases. J Neurosurg 1997; 86(5):793–800.
15. Kleihues P, Cavenee WK, International Agency for Research on Cancer. Pathology and genetics of tumours of the nervous system. World Health Organization classification of tumours. Lyon (France): IARC Press; 2000. p. 314.
16. Louis DN, International Agency for Research on Cancer., and World Health Organization. WHO classification of tumours of the central nervous system. World Health Organization classification of

tumours. 4th edition. Lyon (France): International Agency for Research on Cancer; 2007. p. 309.

17. Perry A, Stafford SL, Scheithauer BW, et al. Meningioma grading: an analysis of histologic parameters. Am J Surg Pathol 1997;21(12):1455–65.

18. Vaubel RA, Chen SG, Raleigh DR, et al. Meningiomas with rhabdoid features lacking other histologic features of malignancy: a study of 44 cases and review of the literature. J Neuropathol Exp Neurol 2016;75(1):44–52.

19. Herscovici Z, Rappaport Z, Sulkes J, et al. Natural history of conservatively treated meningiomas. Neurology 2004;63(6):1133–4.

20. Sahm F, Schrimpf D, Stichel D, et al. DNA methylation-based classification and grading system for meningioma: a multicentre, retrospective analysis. Lancet Oncol 2017;18(5):682–94.

21. Patel AJ, Wan YW, Al-Ouran R, et al. Molecular profiling predicts meningioma recurrence and reveals loss of DREAM complex repression in aggressive tumors. bioRxiv 2019;679480.

22. Vasudevan HN, Braunstein SE, Phillips JJ, et al. Comprehensive molecular profiling identifies FOXM1 as a key transcription factor for meningioma proliferation. Cell Rep 2018;22(13):3672–83.

23. Collord G, Tarpey P, Kurbatova N, et al. An integrated genomic analysis of anaplastic meningioma identifies prognostic molecular signatures. Sci Rep 2018;8(1):13537.

24. Aizer AA, Abedalthagafi M, Bi WL, et al. A prognostic cytogenetic scoring system to guide the adjuvant management of patients with atypical meningioma. Neuro Oncol 2016;18(2):269–74.

25. Al-Mefty O, Kadri PAS, Pravdenkova S, et al. Malignant progression in meningioma: documentation of a series and analysis of cytogenetic findings. J Neurosurg 2004;101(2):210–8.

26. Bi WL, Greenwald NF, Abedalthagafi M, et al. Genomic landscape of high-grade meningiomas. NPJ Genom Med 2017;2.

27. Lee Y, Liu J, Patel S, et al. Genomic landscape of meningiomas. Brain Pathol 2010;20(4):751–62.

28. Mawrin C, Perry A. Pathological classification and molecular genetics of meningiomas. J Neurooncol 2010;99(3):379–91.

29. Zack TI, Schumacher SE, Carter SL, et al. Pan-cancer patterns of somatic copy number alteration. Nat Genet 2013;45(10):1134–40.

30. Zang KD. Meningioma: a cytogenetic model of a complex benign human tumor, including data on 394 karyotyped cases. Cytogenet Cell Genet 2001;93(3–4):207–20.

31. Ruttledge MH, Sarrazin J, Rangaratnam S, et al. Evidence for the complete inactivation of the NF2 gene in the majority of sporadic meningiomas. Nat Genet 1994;6(2):180–4.

32. Abedalthagafi MS, Merrill PH, Bi WL, et al. Angiomatous meningiomas have a distinct genetic profile with multiple chromosomal polysomies including polysomy of chromosome 5. Oncotarget 2014; 5(21):10596–606.

33. Lamszus K, Kluwe L, Matschke J, et al. Allelic losses at 1p, 9q, 10q, 14q, and 22q in the progression of aggressive meningiomas and undifferentiated meningeal sarcomas. Cancer Genet Cytogenet 1999;110(2):103–10.

34. Perry A, Banerjee R, Lohse CM, et al. A role for chromosome 9p21 deletions in the malignant progression of meningiomas and the prognosis of anaplastic meningiomas. Brain Pathol 2002;12(2): 183–90.

35. Bostrom J, Meyer-Puttlitz B, Wolter M, et al. Alterations of the tumor suppressor genes CDKN2A (p16(INK4a)), p14(ARF), CDKN2B (p15(INK4b)), and CDKN2C (p18(INK4c)) in atypical and anaplastic meningiomas. Am J Pathol 2001; 159(2):661–9.

36. Cai DX, James CD, Scheithauer BW, et al. PS6K amplification characterizes a small subset of anaplastic meningiomas. Am J Clin Pathol 2001; 115(2):213–8.

37. Smith MJ, O'Sullivan J, Bhaskar SS, et al. Loss-of-function mutations in SMARCE1 cause an inherited disorder of multiple spinal meningiomas. Nat Genet 2013;45(3):295–8.

38. Smith MJ, Wallace AJ, Bennett C, et al. Germline SMARCE1 mutations predispose to both spinal and cranial clear cell meningiomas. J Pathol 2014;234(4):436–40.

39. Smith MJ, Ahn S, Lee J-I, et al. SMARCE1 mutation screening in classification of clear cell meningiomas. Histopathology 2017;70(5):814–20.

40. Steilen-Gimbel H, Niedermayer I, Feiden W, et al. Unbalanced translocation t(1;3)(p12-13;q11) in meningiomas as the unique feature of chordoid differentiation. Genes Chromosomes Cancer 1999; 26(3):270–2.

41. Shankar GM, Abedalthagafi M, Vaubel RA, et al. Germline and somatic BAP1 mutations in high-grade rhabdoid meningiomas. Neuro Oncol 2017; 19(4):535–45.

42. Shankar GM, Santagata S. BAP1 mutations in high-grade meningioma: implications for patient care. Neuro Oncol 2017;19(11):1447–56.

43. Abdel-Rahman MH, Pilarski R, Cebulla CM, et al. Germline BAP1 mutation predisposes to uveal melanoma, lung adenocarcinoma, meningioma, and other cancers. J Med Genet 2011;48(12):856–9.

44. Wu YT, Ho JT, Lin YJ, et al. Rhabdoid papillary meningioma: a clinicopathologic case series study. Neuropathology 2011;31(6):599–605.

45. Biczok A, Kraus T, Suchorska B, et al. TERT promoter mutation is associated with worse prognosis

in WHO grade II and III meningiomas. J Neurooncol 2018;139(3):671–8.

46. Goutagny S, Nault JC, Mallet M, et al. High incidence of activating TERT promoter mutations in meningiomas undergoing malignant progression. Brain Pathol 2014;24(2):184–9.

47. Sahm F, Schrimpf D, Olar A, et al. TERT promoter mutations and risk of recurrence in meningioma. J Natl Cancer Inst 2016;108(5).

48. Agnihotri S, Suppiah S, Tonge PD, et al. Therapeutic radiation for childhood cancer drives structural aberrations of NF2 in meningiomas. Nat Commun 2017;8(1):186.

49. Harmanci AS, Youngblood MW, Clark VE, et al. Integrated genomic analyses of de novo pathways underlying atypical meningiomas. Nat Commun 2017;8:14433.

50. Fontaine B, Rouleau GA, Seizinger BR, et al. Molecular genetics of neurofibromatosis 2 and related tumors (acoustic neuroma and meningioma). Ann N Y Acad Sci 1991;615:338–43.

51. Lekanne Deprez RH, Bianchi AB, Groen NA, et al. Frequent NF2 gene transcript mutations in sporadic meningiomas and vestibular schwannomas. Am J Hum Genet 1994;54(6):1022–9.

52. Wellenreuther R, Kraus JA, Lenartz D, et al. Analysis of the neurofibromatosis 2 gene reveals molecular variants of meningioma. Am J Pathol 1995; 146(4):827–32.

53. Hartmann C, Sieberns J, Gehlhaar C, et al. NF2 mutations in secretory and other rare variants of meningiomas. Brain Pathol 2006;16(1):15–9.

54. Kros J, de Greve K, van Tilborg A, et al. NF2 status of meningiomas is associated with tumour localization and histology. J Pathol 2001;194(3): 367–72.

55. Perry A, Scheithauer BW, Stafford SL, et al. "Malignancy" in meningiomas: a clinicopathologic study of 116 patients, with grading implications. Cancer 1999;85(9):2046–56.

56. Brastianos PK, Horowitz PM, Santagata S, et al. Genomic sequencing of meningiomas identifies oncogenic SMO and AKT1 mutations. Nat Genet 2013;45(3):285–9.

57. Clark VE, Erson-Omay EZ, Serin A, et al. Genomic analysis of non-NF2 meningiomas reveals mutations in TRAF7, KLF4, AKT1, and SMO. Science 2013;339(6123):1077–80.

58. Sahm F, Bissel J, Koelsche C, et al. AKT1E17K mutations cluster with meningothelial and transitional meningiomas and can be detected by SFRP1 immunohistochemistry. Acta Neuropathol 2013; 126(5):757–62.

59. Reuss DE, Piro RM, Jones DTW, et al. Secretory meningiomas are defined by combined KLF4 K409Q and TRAF7 mutations. Acta Neuropathol 2013;125(3):351–8.

60. Clark VE, Harmanci AS, Bai H, et al. Recurrent somatic mutations in POLR2A define a distinct subset of meningiomas. Nat Genet 2016;48(10):1253–9.

61. Karakas B, Bachman KE, Park BH. Mutation of the PIK3CA oncogene in human cancers. Br J Cancer 2006;94(4):455–9.

62. Yuzawa S, Nishihara H, Tanaka S. Genetic landscape of meningioma. Brain Tumor Pathol 2016;33(4):237–47.

63. Abedalthagafi M, Bi WL, Aizer AA, et al. Oncogenic PI3K mutations are as common as AKT1 and SMO mutations in meningioma. Neuro Oncol 2016;18(5): 649–55.

64. Gao F, Shi L, Russin J, et al. DNA methylation in the malignant transformation of meningiomas. PLoS One 2013;8(1):e54114.

65. Bello MJ, Aminoso C, Lopez-Marin I, et al. DNA methylation of multiple promoter-associated CpG islands in meningiomas: relationship with the allelic status at 1p and 22q. Acta Neuropathol 2004; 108(5):413–21.

66. Olar A, Wani KM, Wilson CD, et al. Global epigenetic profiling identifies methylation subgroups associated with recurrence-free survival in meningioma. Acta Neuropathol 2017;133(3):431–44.

67. Boulagnon-Rombi C, Fleury C, Fichel C, et al. Immunohistochemical approach to the differential diagnosis of meningiomas and their mimics. J Neuropathol Exp Neurol 2017;76(4):289–98.

68. Menke JR, Raleigh DR, Gown AM, et al. Somatostatin receptor 2a is a more sensitive diagnostic marker of meningioma than epithelial membrane antigen. Acta Neuropathol 2015;130(3):441–3.

69. Carroll RS, Glowacka D, Dashner K, et al. Progesterone receptor expression in meningiomas. Cancer Res 1993;53(6):1312–6.

70. Du Z, Brewster R, Merrill PH, et al. Meningioma transcription factors link cell lineage with systemic metabolic cues. Neuro Oncol 2018;20(10):1331–43.

71. Rossi ML, Cruz Sanchez F, Hughes JT, et al. Immunocytochemical study of the cellular immune response in meningiomas. J Clin Pathol 1988;41(3):314–9.

72. Asai J, Suzuki R, Fujimoto T, et al. Fluorescence automatic cell sorter and immunohistochemical investigation of CD68-positive cells in meningioma. Clin Neurol Neurosurg 1999;101(4):229–34.

73. Domingues P, Gonzalez-Tablas M, Otero A, et al. Tumor infiltrating immune cells in gliomas and meningiomas. Brain Behav Immun 2016;53:1–15.

74. Domingues PH, Teodosio C, Ortiz J, et al. Immunophenotypic identification and characterization of tumor cells and infiltrating cell populations in meningiomas. The American Journal of Pathology 2012;181(5):1749–61.

75. Domingues PH, Teodosio C, Otero A, et al. Association between inflammatory infiltrates and isolated monosomy 22/del(22q) in meningiomas. PLoS One 2013;8(10):e74798.

76. Pinton L, Solito S, Masetto E, et al. Immunosuppressive activity of tumor-infiltrating myeloid cells in patients with meningioma. Oncoimmunology 2018;7(7):e1440931.

77. Grund S, Schittenhelm J, Roser F, et al. The microglial/macrophagic response at the tumour-brain border of invasive meningiomas. Neuropathol Appl Neurobiol 2009;35(1):82–8.

78. Han SJ, Reis G, Kohanbash G, et al. Expression and prognostic impact of immune modulatory molecule PD-L1 in meningioma. J Neurooncol 2016;130(3):543–52.

79. Du Z, Abedalthagafi M, Aizer AA, et al. Increased expression of the immune modulatory molecule PD-L1 (CD274) in anaplastic meningioma. Oncotarget 2015;6(7):4704–16.

80. Fang L, Lowther DE, Meizlish ML, et al. The immune cell infiltrate populating meningiomas is composed of mature, antigen-experienced T and B cells. Neuro Oncol 2013;15(11):1479–90.

81. Proctor DT, Patel Z, Lama S, et al. Identification of PD-L2, B7-H3 and CTLA-4 immune checkpoint proteins in genetic subtypes of meningioma. Oncoimmunology 2019;8(1):e1512943.

82. Viaene AN, Zhang B, Martinez-Lage M, et al. Transcriptome signatures associated with meningioma progression. Acta Neuropathol Commun 2019; 7(1):67.

83. Suppiah S, Agnihotri S, Liu J, et al. GENE-37. Pathway analysis of radiation-induced meningiomas reveals that tumours with NF2-fusion have upregulation of inflammatory pathways. Neuro-Oncology 2017;19(suppl_6):vi100.

84. Suppiah S, Liu J, Mamatjan Y, et al. 56 unique immune microenvironment in NF2-fusion positive radiation induced meningiomas. Canadian Journal of Neurological Sciences / Journal Canadien des Sciences Neurologiques 2018;45(S3):S17.

85. Suppiah S, Karimi S, Mamatjan Y, et al. TMIC-17. Immune microenvironment of NF2-altered radiation-induced meningiomas. Neuro-Oncology 2018;20(suppl_6):vi259.

86. Zador Z, Landry AP, Balas M, et al. Skull base meningiomas have a distinct immune landscape. bioRxiv 2019;525444.

87. Fletcher CDM, World Health Organization, International Agency for Research on Cancer. WHO classification of tumours of soft tissue and bone. World Health Organization classification of tumours. 4th edition. Lyon (France): IARC Press; 2013. p. 468.

88. Mena H, Ribas JL, Pezeshkpour GH, et al. Hemangiopericytoma of the central nervous system: a review of 94 cases. Hum Pathol 1991;22(1):84–91.

89. Schiariti M, Goetz P, El-Maghraby H, et al. Hemangiopericytoma: long-term outcome revisited. Clinical article. J Neurosurg 2011;114(3):747–55.

90. Gengler C, Guillou L. Solitary fibrous tumour and haemangiopericytoma: evolution of a concept. Histopathology 2006;48(1):63–74.

91. Gold JS, Antonescu CR, Hajdu C, et al. Clinicopathologic correlates of solitary fibrous tumors. Cancer 2002;94(4):1057–68.

92. Bouvier C, Metellus P, Maues de Paula A, et al. Solitary fibrous tumors and hemangiopericytomas of the meninges: overlapping pathological features and common prognostic factors suggest the same spectrum of tumors. Brain Pathol 2012; 22(4):511–21.

93. Demicco EG, Park MS, Araujo DM, et al. Solitary fibrous tumor: a clinicopathological study of 110 cases and proposed risk assessment model. Mod Pathol 2012;25(9):1298–306.

94. Robinson DR, Wu YM, Kalyana-Sundaram S, et al. Identification of recurrent NAB2-STAT6 gene fusions in solitary fibrous tumor by integrative sequencing. Nat Genet 2013;45(2):180–5.

95. Chmielecki J, Crago AM, Rosenberg M, et al. Whole-exome sequencing identifies a recurrent NAB2-STAT6 fusion in solitary fibrous tumors. Nat Genet 2013;45(2):131–2.

96. Mohajeri A, Tayebwa J, Collin A, et al. Comprehensive genetic analysis identifies a pathognomonic NAB2/STAT6 fusion gene, nonrandom secondary genomic imbalances, and a characteristic gene expression profile in solitary fibrous tumor. Genes Chromosomes Cancer 2013;52(10):873–86.

97. Doyle LA, Vivero M, Dm Fletcher C, et al. Nuclear expression of STAT6 distinguishes solitary fibrous tumor from histologic mimics. Mod Pathol 2014; 27(3):390–5.

98. Olson NJ, Linos K. Dedifferentiated solitary fibrous tumor: a concise review. Arch Pathol Lab Med 2018;142(6):761–6.

99. Barthelmess S, Geddert H, Boltze C, et al. Solitary fibrous tumors/hemangiopericytomas with different variants of the NAB2-STAT6 gene fusion are characterized by specific histomorphology and distinct clinicopathological features. Am J Pathol 2014; 184(4):1209–18.

100. Yuzawa S, Nishihara H, Wang L, et al. Analysis of NAB2-STAT6 gene fusion in 17 cases of meningeal solitary fibrous tumor/hemangiopericytoma: review of the literature. Am J Surg Pathol 2016;40(8): 1031–40.

101. Akaike K, Kurisaki-Arakawa A, Hara K, et al. Distinct clinicopathological features of NAB2-STAT6 fusion gene variants in solitary fibrous tumor with emphasis on the acquisition of highly malignant potential. Hum Pathol 2015;46(3): 347–56.

102. Bahrami A, Lee S, Shaefer IM, et al. TERT promoter mutations and prognosis in solitary fibrous tumor. Mod Pathol 2016;29(12):1511–22.

Sellar Tumors

Katherine E. Schwetye, MD, PhD[a], Sonika M. Dahiya, MBBS, MD[b],*

KEYWORDS

- Sella • Pituitary • Adenoma • Hypophysitis • Craniopharyngioma • IgG4 • Pituicytoma
- Neurohypophysis

Key points

- Complex sellar anatomy results in a wide spectrum of neoplastic and non-neoplastic entities, including autoimmune processes and secondary involvement by various systemic diseases.
- Magnetic resonance imaging remains a key diagnostic tool.
- Pituitary adenomas are classified according to their developmental lineage (PIT, T-PIT, or SF expression).
- The two histologic variants of craniopharyngioma demonstrate mutually exclusive genetic signatures: *CTNNB1* mutations in adamantinomatous type, and *BRAF V600E mutation* in papillary type.
- Tumors of the posterior pituitary are derived from a common lineage, as all express TTF-1, which can be used as a diagnostic marker.

ABSTRACT

Sellar region lesions include a broad range of benign and malignant neoplastic as well as non-neoplastic entities, many of which are newly described or have recently revised nomenclature. In contrast to other intracranial sites, imaging features are relatively less specific, and the need for histopathological diagnosis is of paramount importance. This review will describe pituitary adenomas, inflammatory lesions, and tumors unique to the region (craniopharyngioma) as well as tumors which may occur in but are not exclusively localized to the sellar location (schwannoma, metastasis, etc.).

PITUITARY ADENOMA

INTRODUCTORY PARAGRAPH

Pituitary adenomas predominantly affect adult men and women in the third to sixth decades, although they occasionally arise in children[1]; rates are higher among Black than White individuals and also higher among Hispanics than non-Hispanics.[2,3] Symptoms reflect local mass effect, including headache, visual deficits, and compression of cavernous sinus structures (notably, cranial nerves III, IV, and VI) as well as hormonal hypersecretion. Hormonal hypersecretion depends on the specific subtype. Elevated prolactin (PRL) levels occur due to "stalk effect," when the mass of a tumor blocks infundibular dopamine release; dopamine inhibits the basally high-secretory tone of lactotrophs, so loss of secretory inhibition results in hyperprolactinemia. Clinical symptoms include amenorrhea and galactorrhea in women and subtle sexual dysfunction and infertility in men. Other hypersecreted hormones result in clinically identifiable phenotypes. A growth hormone (GH)-producing tumor, somatotroph adenoma, yields gigantism before closure of epiphyseal bony plates, acromegaly, soft tissue swelling, hypertension, hyperglycemia, and sleep apnea. An adrenocorticotropic hormone (ACTH)-producing tumor, corticotroph adenoma, causes Cushing disease,

[a] Department of Pathology, Saint Louis University, 1402 South Grand Boulevard, St Louis, MO 63104, USA;
[b] Department of Pathology and Immunology, Washington University in St. Louis, 660 South Euclid Avenue, St Louis, MO 63110, USA
* Corresponding author.
E-mail address: sdahiya@wustl.edu

Surgical Pathology 13 (2020) 305–329
https://doi.org/10.1016/j.path.2020.02.006
1875-9181/20/© 2020 Elsevier Inc. All rights reserved.

surgpath.theclinics.com

with elevated cortisol levels leading to central obesity, skin striae, hyperglycemia, osteoporosis, and hirsutism. Tumors secreting follicle stimulating hormone (FSH) and/or luteinizing hormone (LH), gonadotroph adenomas, are usually clinically silent due to the low serum levels of hormone. Thyroid-stimulating hormone (TSH)-producing tumors, thyrotroph adenomas, may cause hyperthyroidism or may arise in the setting of hypothyroidism. Overall, metastasis is rare. When present, either in cerebrospinal or systemic locations, the tumor is designated as pituitary carcinoma. No single set of histologic features is known to accurately predict the metastatic potential of a pituitary adenoma. There is no World Health Organization (WHO) grade assigned to pituitary adenomas in the current system (WHO 2017[4]); the prior version (WHO 2004[5]) suggested the designation of "atypical" based on p53 overexpression and Ki-67 indices, but this is no longer recommended. Instead, pituitary adenomas should be assessed for proliferation (mitotic count and Ki-67 index), tumor invasion, and functional status, features associated with aggressive clinical behavior.[6–9]

The 2017 revision of the WHO classification system of pituitary adenomas also introduced the concept of lineage-specific categorization, as opposed to categorization by the standalone expression of hormones. Three main transcription factors define the categories: PIT-1 (pituitary-specific POU-class homeodomain transcription factor, for differentiation of somatotrophs, lactotrophs, and thyrotrophs); SF-1 (steroidogenic factor 1, regulating gonadotroph cell differentiation), and T-PIT (T-box family member TBX19 transcription factor, for differentiation of corticotrophs).[4]

There is a spectrum of clinically silent to "functional" (hypersecretory) tumors among pituitary adenomas. Serum levels of hormone may not parallel the physical size of the tumor and also, immunohistochemical reactivity does not always reflect the functional status of the tumor.

GROSS FEATURES

MRI is the preferred modality to identify lesions within the pituitary gland and surrounding parasellar region and provides high accuracy.[10] The normal anterior pituitary gland is isointense to gray matter on noncontrast T1- and T2-weighted sequences. The posterior pituitary has intrinsic high T1 signal but is hypointense on T2. The infundibulum and gland progressively enhance with contrast, whereas contrast uptake by pituitary adenomas is slower. Although most of them are solid

and enhancing (**Fig. 1**A), they can be sometimes be cystic.

There are two main clinico-radiological grading systems to describe invasion of pituitary adenomas. The Hardy system (1976[11]) grades adenomas by imaging features. Grade I includes microadenomas, intrapituitary lesions less than 1 cm in diameter; grade II describes macroadenomas at least 1 cm in diameter; grade III tumors are locally invasive, causing bony erosion of sella turcica; and grade IV macroadenomas invade extrasellar structures such as bone, hypothalamus, and cavernous sinus. The term "giant pituitary adenoma" is generally reserved for lesions greater than 4 cm in size. The Knosp system (1993[12]) is based on involvement of spaces defined by a medial tangent, the intercarotid line, and a lateral tangent on the intra- and supracavernous internal carotid arteries. Grade 0 represents the normal condition, and grade 4 corresponds to the total encasement of the intracavernous carotid artery. In the original study, most grade 2 and all grades 3 and 4 lesions showed intraoperative evidence of invasion of the cavernous sinus.

Cavernous sinus invasion (CSI) is the most common and significant risk factor for incomplete surgical resection,[13–16] with Knosp grades 3 or 4 all showing CSI.[17] However, because of the imprecision of neuroimaging, intraoperative, and histopathologic evaluation, invasion is not currently part of the formal grading scheme in the most recent WHO classification system.[4]

Grossly, adenomas are soft lesions with a tan-brown discoloration. Microadenomas may be difficult for both surgeon and pathologist to identify grossly.

MICROSCOPIC FEATURES

In contrast to polymorphous cell population of adenohypophyseal tissue arranged in acinar architecture (**Fig. 1**B, C), adenoma is monomorphic with loss of normal acinar architecture (**Fig. 1**D, E). As other neuroendocrine tumors, pituitary adenomas show a multitude of architectural arrangements: diffuse sheets of relatively monomorphic cells, as well as papillary and trabecular patterns. Small mucin-filled cysts found frequently in gonadotroph adenomas as well as other cytologic variants may occasionally pose a diagnostic challenge, especially in small biopsies. Cytologically, tumor cells may be acidophilic, basophilic, or chromophobic. In most cases, the histomorphologic appearance as a standalone is insufficient to subtype the adenoma (see "Diagnosis").

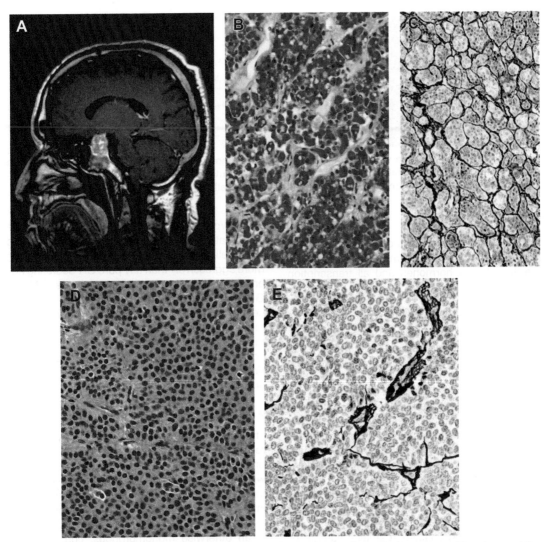

Fig. 1. Contrast-enhancing sellar mass in an adult (*A*). Polymorphous cell population arranged in acinar architecture in adenohypophyseal gland (*B*). Reticulin further accentuates the normal acinar arrangement of normal cells (*C*). The neoplastic cells in adenoma are uniform and monomorphous (*D*) and demonstrate loss of normal acinar architecture as highlighted by a reticulin stain (*E*).

DIFFERENTIAL DIAGNOSIS

Pituitary adenomas may exhibit challenging morphologic features, including clear cell change similar to oligodendroglioma, perivascular pseudorosette architecture similar to ependymoma, pseudopapillary pattern, or nuclear enlargement and hyperchromasia. Fibrosis and small cell–like morphology in some tumors, often following dopamine agonist treatment, can pose diagnostic dilemmas.

DIAGNOSIS

Gonadotroph Adenoma

Gonadotroph adenomas are usually clinically nonfunctioning, indolent tumors found in older adults. Histologically, most are cytologically bland and are arranged in a perivascular or patternless architecture (**Fig. 2**A). Small cysts can sometimes be interspersed.

Positive SF1 immunostaining is sufficient to diagnose gonadotroph adenoma.[18] FSH and LH show patchy or focal reactivity (**Fig. 2**B, C, respectively). Keratin expression may be focal or diffuse.

Hormone-Negative Adenoma (Formerly Null Cell Adenoma)

These tumors are likewise SF1 immunopositive and are histologically similar to gonadotroph adenomas, without FSH or LH reactivity.

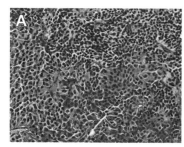
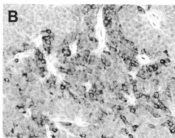
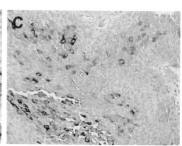

Fig. 2. Gonadotroph adenoma with a biphasic population of tumor cells constituted by a subset of cells with moderate amounts of eosinophilic cytoplasm to the others with scant vacuolated to negligible cytoplasm (*A*). Follicle stimulating hormone (*B*) and luteinizing hormone (*C*) are focally expressed within the tumor cells.

Null Cell Adenoma

A true null cell adenoma, as defined by the 2017 WHO classification[19] is immunonegative for all specific pituitary hormones and all transcription factors.

Growth Hormone Adenoma

The PIT1-driven GH-producing adenomas typically present with clinical symptoms. Two subtypes are based on the electron microscopic features: densely granulated and sparsely granulated.

The densely granulated variant shows a diffuse growth pattern, monotonous cytologic features, and eosinophilic cytoplasm. Immunoreactivity for GH is detectable. Low-molecular-weight keratins fill the cytoplasm. The proliferative index is low, and they are typically macroadenomas.

An "intermediate/mixed/transitional" subtype of GH adenoma has been described, as determined by perinuclear CAM5.2 immunostaining that fills the cytoplasm and contains a smaller number of admixed cells with fibrous bodies or intermediate forms of keratin accumulation.[20] Clinically, these forms respond similarly to somatostatin analogues as the densely granulated variant.

Sparsely granulated GH tumors show a diffuse growth pattern, significant cellular pleomorphism, eccentrically placed nuclei, and paranuclear clearing. The characteristic "fibrous bodies" may be detected on routine stains as pale eosinophilic paranuclear structures (**Fig. 3**A) but are highlighted best by Cam 5.2 immunostaining (**Fig. 3**B). Immunostaining for GH is weak (**Fig.** 3C) or negative. Although the proliferative index may be low, it is a more clinically aggressive subtype as compared with the densely granulated variant.[21]

Mixed Growth Hormone/Prolactin-Secreting Adenoma

These PIT-1-driven, GH-secreting tumors can be subdivided into 3 morphologic types: the mixed GH cell/prolactin (PRL) cell adenoma, the mammosomatotroph cell adenoma, and the acidophilic stem cell adenoma; these mixed tumors behave more aggressively than any pure GH-secreting adenomas, with a lower surgical cure rate.[22] Mixed GH/PRL adenomas are composed of 2 distinct cell types, each of which expresses a unique hormone, as compared with the monocellular mammosomatotroph cell adenomas in which cells coexpress GH and PRL. The distinction is predominantly considered to be clinically unimportant.

Acidophilic Stem Cell Adenoma

This subtype of mixed adenoma is very rare and represents only the minority of GH/PRL-producing tumors.[22,23] Most patients present with symptoms of hyperprolactinemia, and most tumors are rapidly growing macroadenomas with invasive features. Histologically, acidophilic stem cell adenomas show large cytoplasmic vacuoles in an otherwise monomorphous, chromophobic to slightly acidophilic cytoplasm. Oncocytic change with the presence of giant mitochondria is characteristic. Immunoreactivity for PRL and, to a lesser extent, GH is present in the cytoplasm of the same tumor cells. Electron microscopy shows a single, immature population with features of sparsely granulated GH adenoma subtype but contains fewer fibrous bodies. Low serum levels of PRL correspond to their poor response to standard therapies.

Prolactin-Secreting Adenoma

Another, typically clinically functional, PIT1-driven tumor is the prolactinoma (lactotroph adenoma). Most are sparsely granulated, with only rare examples being densely granulated. Prolactinoma in men is associated with aggressive clinical behavior. These tumors usually demonstrate sheeted or interrupted trabecular growth patterns, and more prominent nucleoli, and

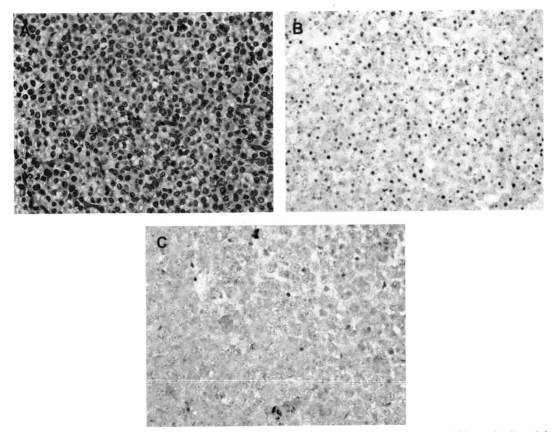

Fig. 3. Sparsely granulated somatotroph adenoma characterized by pale intracytoplasmic "fibrous bodies" (*A*) that are strongly immunoreactive with CAM 5.2 (*B*) and show overall weak expression of growth hormone (*C*).

amphophilic cytoplasm as compared with many other subtypes (**Fig. 4**A). **Fig. 4**B shows an example of PRL immunoreactivity in a diffuse pattern. Depending on the time course of treatment, dopamine agonists may cause dense fibrosis and a "small blue cell" appearance due to apoptosis[24,25] (**Fig. 5**).

Corticotroph Adenoma

TPIT-driven corticotroph adenomas also are subtyped into densely and sparsely granulated. The typical "microadenoma" is a densely granulated ACTH adenoma composed of sheets of monotonous round cells, with abundant basophilic, PAS-positive cytoplasm and strong diffuse immunoreactivity for ACTH (**Fig. 6**). Sparsely granulated ACTH adenomas are more chromophobic, weakly PAS-positive, with less cytoplasmic volume, with more focal ACTH immunoreactivity. The sparsely granulated ACTH adenoma more often is a clinically silent, large, invasive tumor. Slightly confusing is the categorization of 2 silent variants: basophilic, densely granulated (silent type 1) and chromophobic, sparsely granulated (silent type 2).

Crooke cell adenoma is an uncommon variant of ACTH-immunoreactive adenoma in which tumor cells show ringlike, cytokeratin-positive accumulations, to be distinguished from the more common Crooke cell change in adjacent nonadenomatous anterior pituitary gland; Crooke cell change indicates the clinical condition of functional hypercortisolemia. Keratin stain highlights these features.

Corticotroph hyperplasia rarely causes Cushing syndrome and should be carefully evaluated by reticulin stain. A true microadenoma will demonstrate complete loss of acinar architecture. ACTH immunohistochemistry is also necessary.

Thyroid-Stimulating Hormone–Producing Adenoma

Very rarely (~2% of all pituitary adenomas[26]), these PIT1-driven invasive macroadenomas grow in a diffuse pattern with frequent perivascular pseudorosettes. Nuclear pleomorphism and spindled morphology are more common. Extensive fibrosis may be seen. TSH and α-SU are variably immunoreactive.[26,27]

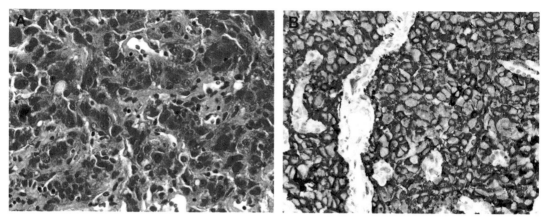

Fig. 4. Prolactinoma. Note the prominent nucleoli, which is a frequent finding in this subtype (*A*). Diffuse and strong reactivity for prolactin in a densely granulated example (*B*).

Plurihormonal PIT1-Positive Adenoma

Previously designated as "silent adenoma subtype 3," the plurihormonal PIT1-positive adenomas are rare tumors, which clinically present with mass effect or signs of hyperthyroidism, acromegaly or galactorrhea, and amenorrhea and are important to recognize given their aggressive clinical behavior.[28] Histologically, they are composed of elongate cells with nuclear spheridia on electron microscopy and show reactivity to GH, PRL, TSH, and α-SU.[26]

Pituitary Apoplexy

Apoplexy describes the clinical situation when hemorrhagic infarction occurs in the sellar region, typically in the setting of pituitary macroadenoma, and sometimes in the post-partum period as a result of physiologic hyperplasia. Sudden-onset symptoms include headache, cranial nerve palsy, or visual disturbances. Histologically, hemorrhagic infarction characterized by ghost outlines of necrotic cells is readily seen (**Fig. 7**A). Reticulin highlights the loss of normal acinar architecture in adenoma (**Fig. 7**B) and its preservation in normal adenohypophyses, and depending on the age of the infarction, tumor cells may retain antigenicity and show reactivity with neuroendocrine markers, ie, synaptophysin and chromogranin (**Fig. 7**C), and keratins, and pituitary hormones.

Mixed Pituitary Adenoma-Gangliocytoma

This tumor, generally considered to represent neuronal metaplasia of adenoma cells, shows a variety of histologic patterns, although the clinical, neuroimaging, and intraoperative presentation is that of a pituitary adenoma without any prognostic connotation. Notably, it harbors large dysmorphic ganglionic cells (**Fig. 8**) that are frequently reactive with neuronal markers and negative with glial markers. The two components may be sharply demarcated or variably admixed with predominance of adenoma. Transitional tumor cells or mature ganglion cells may be immunoreactive for pituitary hormones or transcription factors, consistent with a metaplastic process rather than a "collision tumor."[29]

PROGNOSIS

Both medical and surgical approaches are used for the management of pituitary adenoma,

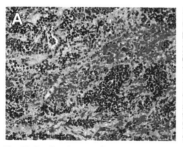
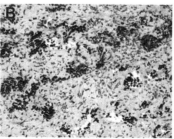
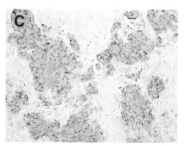

Fig. 5. Prolactinoma from a patient who was medically treated with carbegoline demonstrating "small cells" with minimal cytoplasm, high nuclear-cytoplasmic ratio, and hyperchromatic nuclei (*A*) as well as stromal fibrosis (*B*). Punctate staining pattern seen with prolactin (*C*).

Fig. 6. Densely granulated ACTH-secreting adenoma that is strongly immunoreactive with ACTH.

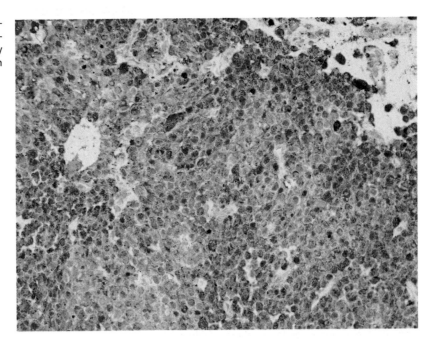

depending on the subtype. Most prolactinomas respond to dopamine receptor agonists, particularly those with hypersecretion of prolactin. Somatotroph adenomas are treated with somatostatin analogues (octreotide), and in the case of sparsely granulated subtypes, GH receptor antagonist (GHRH) antagonists are an adjuvant therapy.

Surgical management, including transsphenoidal/translabial and endoscopic transnasal approaches, aims to resect as much tumor as possible. For intrasellar tumors, the transsphenoidal or endonasal endoscopic techniques show similar results but for larger extrasellar tumors the endonasal approach may be preferred. A transfrontal approach may be required to decompress the visual pathways for larger tumors.

Complications of surgery include cerebrospinal fluid (CSF) leak, residual tumor, postoperative diabetes insipidus, and apoplexy in residual adenoma.

If a resection is subtotal, outcome is also related to any residual hypersecretory endocrinopathy.

Determination of subtype helps both prognosticate and predict response to therapy. Well-differentiated adenomas respond better, such as prolactinomas with dopamine agonists and densely granulated GH adenomas with somatostatin analogues. In the case of the sparsely granulated GH adenomas, a switch from somatostatin analogue to GHRH, or addition of GHRH, may show improved response.

Conventional radiation or radiosurgery is considered for recurrent and/or invasive, aggressive adenomas; subtyping does not necessarily mandate the use of radiation.

OVERVIEW: MOLECULAR PATHOLOGY OF PITUITARY ADENOMAS

Pituitary adenomas are most commonly sporadic, and in most, the primary genetic defect is

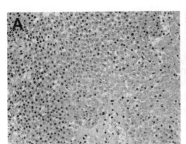
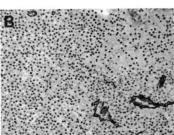
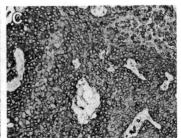

Fig. 7. Large areas of necrosis, characterized by "ghost outlines" of tumor cells, are pathognomic of apoplexy (*A*). Lack of normal acinar architecture is supported by a reticulin stain (*B*). There is strong and diffuse chromogranin immunoreactivity despite extensive necrosis, which suggests preserved antigenicity in a subset of apoplectic cases (*C*).

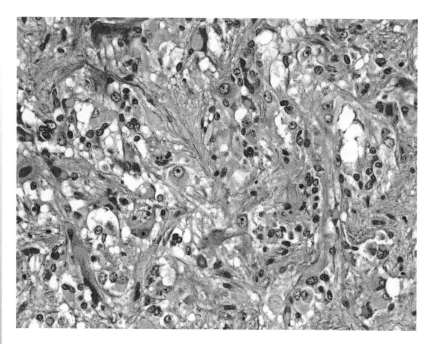

Fig. 8. Neuronal differentiation is an unusual phenomenon in pituitary adenoma. Several dysmorphic neuronal elements, including some large forms akin to ganglion cells, are seen.

unknown. Somatic mutations in the *GNAS* gene are found in 40% of somatotroph adenomas, 10% of clinically nonfunctioning pituitary adenomas, and in 5% of corticotroph adenomas.[30–32] Nonsyndromic gigantism has been related to inactivating germline mutations on the AIP gene and more recently to germline or somatic duplication of the *GPR101* gene.[33–35] Mutations in the *USP8* gene are identified in 36% to 62% of sporadic corticotroph adenomas.[30–32]

Other oncogenes and tumor suppressor genes that have been shown to be linked to pituitary tumorigenesis, progression, and malignant transformation include the oncogene pituitary tumor-transforming gene, the protooncogene *H-ras*, and the tumor suppressor genes *RB* and *TP53*.[30–32]

ASSOCIATED GENETIC CHANGES/ ALTERATIONS

Although most pituitary adenomas are sporadic, some well-known hereditary conditions are associated with pituitary adenomas: multiple endocrine neoplasias 1 and 4 (MEN1 and MEN4); the Carney complex, related to mutations of the tumor suppressor gene *PRKAR1A*; McCune-Albright syndrome, related to activating mutation of the gsp oncogene; SDH-related hereditary pheochromocytoma/paraganglioma syndrome; isolated familial somatotrophinoma (IFS), associated with a loss of heterozygosity at the 11q13 locus but not with the *MEN1* gene; familial isolated pituitary

adenoma (FIPA) syndrome; and X-linked acrogigantism (XLAG), associated with GPR101 microduplication. The syndromic tumors tend to be somatotroph or lactotroph adenomas. In addition, the rare embryonal-like pituitary blastoma occurs in the setting of *DICER1* mutation in infants or young children.[36]

Pathologic Key Features— Pituitary Adenomas

Commonly seen in adults, solid and/or cystic enhancing sellar mass, rarely can be parasellar in ectopic tissue; loss of normal acinar architecture, which can be highlighted by reticulin stain; monomorphic cell population; typically low proliferation indices; acute presentation in patients with apoplexy

Infrequent in children and adolescents with predilection for latter

Current classification based on lineage-specific markers: SF (gonadotroph adenomas), PIT (lactotroph, somatotroph, mixed GH/PRL, TSH-producing, and plurihormonal adenomas), and T-PIT (corticotroph adenomas); lack of hormone or transcription factor expression is designated "null cell adenoma"

Hormone-producing tumors produce clinical symptoms (eg, somatotroph, corticotroph, lactotroph adenomas) versus clinically silent tumors; a spectrum exists

Assess mitotic rate, proliferative activity, and invasion; "atypical" designation (WHO 2004) no longer recommended (WHO 2017)

Clinically more aggressive subtypes include sparsely granulated GH tumors, mixed GH/PRL-secreting adenomas, acidophilic stem cell adenoma, and plurihormonal PIT1-positive adenoma (formerly "silent adenoma subtype 3")

A minority of tumors occur in syndromic settings: MEN1, MEN4, Carney complex, McCune-Albright syndrome, SDH-related hereditary pheochromocytoma/paraganglioma syndrome, IFS, familial isolated pituitary adenoma (FIPA) syndrome, and XLAG; syndromic tumors tend to be GH or PRL adenomas

HYPOPHYSITIS

INTRODUCTION

Hypophysitis, or inflammation of the pituitary gland, describes a spectrum of underlying causes and can generally be classified as primary or secondary; latter can be seen in association with sarcoidosis, Sjogren syndrome, granulomatosis with polyangiitis (GPA; Wegener disease), Langerhans cell histiocytosis (LCH), and Erdheim-Chester disease.

Primary hypophysitis occurs in approximately equal proportions of men and women and is commonly associated with other autoimmune disorders, particularly thyroid disorders (Hashimoto thyroiditis and Grave disease). The most common infiltrate is lymphocytic, and less commonly granulomatous and xanthomatous inflammation may be seen. Secondary causes of granulomatous hypophysitis include tuberculosis, sarcoidosis, syphilis, LCH, GPA, and Rathke Cleft Cyst (RC) rupture.

In the new era of checkpoint inhibitor and other immune therapies, there is an emerging class of immunotherapy-associated hypophysitis, which often presents with headache and anterior hypopituitarism.[37] The degree of pituitary enlargement is typically mild, and compression of the optic apparatus is very rare. Unlike other forms of hypophysitis, diabetes insipidus is unusual in patients with immunotherapy-associated hypophysitis. Of note, no case of immunotherapy-associated hypophysitis has been confirmed by pituitary gland biopsy.[37]

Reversible or irreversible hypopituitarism may be a rare side effect following treatment with interferon-α, and interferon-α/ribavirin combination therapy has been associated with cases of granulomatous hypophysitis with anterior pituitary dysfunction.[38] Very recently, the antiinterleukin-12, and -23 monoclonal antibody ustekinumab (in treatment of psoriasis) has been associated with a case of hypophysitis with panhypopituitarism.[39]

GROSS FEATURES

Because the inflammatory infiltrate typically presents as a mass lesion, imaging studies may suggest pituitary adenoma due to homogeneous contrast-enhancement (**Fig. 9**A), and the patient is referred for surgery. Intraoperative diagnosis by touch or smear preparations and frozen section dictates the extent of resection, which would be undertaken for decompressive measures.

MICROSCOPIC FEATURES

Lymphocytic hypophysitis is an infiltration of the anterior pituitary by lymphocytes, including reactive follicles, plasma cells, and variable amounts of fibrosis. Necrosis can be either nonspecific or specific for certain cell types. Granulomatous hypophysitis is composed of histiocytes, multinucleated giant cells, and lymphoplasmacytic inflammation (see **Fig. 9**B). Immunostains for neuroendocrine markers, ie, synaptophysin and chromogranin (see **Fig. 9**C), as well as lymphocyte markers (pan-lymphocyte: CD45 {see **Fig. 9**D}; T-cell: CD3; B-cell: CD20), and histiocytic markers aid in characterizing this process further. Xanthomatous inflammation also contains S100- and CD1a-negative histiocytes (predominant), lymphocytes, variable granuloma formation, and acellular eosinophilic debris.

DIFFERENTIAL DIAGNOSIS

The histologic differential diagnosis includes lymphoma, immunoglobulin G4 (IgG4)-related disease (discussed later in this article), infectious process, secondary changes related to a ruptured Rathke cleft cyst, and organization associated with pituitary apoplexy.

DIAGNOSIS

Diagnosis is based on a combination of clinical, imaging, and histopathologic features.

PROGNOSIS

Primary hypophysitis can be self-limiting, and spontaneous remission may occur, although rigorous studies of the disease are lacking given its rarity. Primary hypophysitis frequently evolves

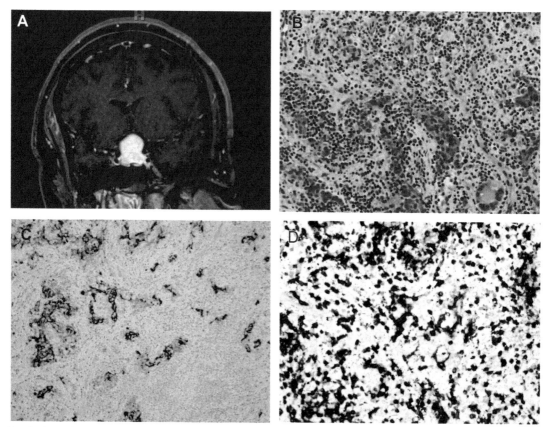

Fig. 9. Granulomatous hypophysitis. Homogeneously solid contrast-enhancing lesion on MRI is usually mistaken for a pituitary adenoma (*A*). Exuberant chronic inflammatory cell infiltrate with invasion of the residual acini along with scattered multinucleate giant cells and fibrosis in the background (*B*). The residual adenohypophyseal tissue can be highlighted by a chromogranin (*C*) or synaptophysin. CD45 stains lymphocytes in the abundant chronic inflammatory cell infiltrate (*D*).

to fibrosis, pituitary atrophy, and may result in "empty sella."[40] Most patients will require long-term hormone replacement. It is unknown whether glucocorticoid treatment is effective. As such, conservative management is recommended for primary hypophysitis unless symptoms are severe and progressive. High-dose glucocorticoids are the first-line treatment to improve the swelling of the pituitary and improve the symptoms related to significant sella compression. The presence of central diabetes insipidus is a poor prognostic factor for response to glucocorticoids. Glucocorticoid therapy is less effective in granulomatous or xanthomatous hypophysitis. In cases of glucocorticoid-resistant hypophysitis, azathioprine, methotrexate, cyclosporine A, and rituximab have been used successfully.[40,41] Surgery is considered only in cases with serious and progressive deficits of the visual field, visual acuity, or nerve paralysis not responsive to medical treatment. Progression/relapse occurs in 11% to 25%

of patients at mean 3-year follow-up.[41] Recovery rates of visual deficits related to chiasmal compression are also low. Finally, stereotactic radiotherapy has been effectively used in selected patients who have failed medical treatment or suffer from repeated recurrence of lymphocytic hypophysitis.[42]

 Pathologic Key Features— Hypophysitis

Primary versus secondary types

Primary hypophysitis often associated with another autoimmune diseases; lymphocytic > granulomatous > xanthomatous

Rare examples associated with checkpoint inhibitor or other targeted therapies

Differential Diagnosis—
Hypophysitis

Pituitary apoplexy

Lymphoma

IgG4-related disease

Infection

IMMUNOGLOBULIN G4 DISEASE: DURAL BASED AND/OR INVOLVEMENT OF PITUITARY GLAND

INTRODUCTION

IgG4-related disease (IgG4-RD), a fibroinflammatory disease that preferentially affects pancreas, salivary gland, the orbit, lymph nodes, lung, and kidney, may also involve the sellar region. It may present as a mass or diffusely infiltrative lesion. IgG4-RD hypophysitis shows a female:male ratio of 2.4:1.[43] Intracranial IgG4-RD presents as pachymeningitis or hypophysitis and generally does not affect the brain parenchyma. When the pituitary gland or stalk is affected, signs include hypopituitarism, diabetes insipidus, or local mass effect.

GROSS FEATURES

There is a wide spectrum of imaging and gross features attributable to IgG4-RD, most of which are nonspecific for the entity. MRI is the modality of choice. Typically, imaging shows an enlargement of the pituitary gland or mass lesion of the pituitary, at times causing optic chiasm compression, thickened pituitary stalk, or mass formation in the infundibulum. Disappearance of physiologic posterior pituitary bright spot on T1-weighed image is also common. Cystic formation in the enlarged anterior pituitary or "empty sella" has also been described, and the diagnosis is often omitted in the radiologic differential, particularly when serum levels of IgG4 are normal.[44]

MICROSCOPIC FEATURES

IgG4-RD is manifest histologically by a lymphoplasmacytic infiltrate with an increased number of plasma cells, predominantly of the IgG4 subtype, storiform fibrosis, and obliterative phlebitis.

DIFFERENTIAL DIAGNOSIS

The differential diagnosis, on imaging and histopathologic examination, includes mass-forming lesions and some immune-mediated diseases (eg, Churg-Strauss syndrome, multicentric Castleman disease, sarcoidosis, Sjogren syndrome). Histopathologic examination should help to establish the diagnosis. Lymphocytic hypophysitis may closely mimic IgG4-RD; although both entities are characterized by a lymphoplasmacytic infiltrate, the latter shows a predominance of plasma cells, whereas the former shows admixed B and T lymphocytes in greater proportion.

DIAGNOSIS

In conjunction with imaging features, a diagnosis of IgG4-RD may be rendered based on the histopathologic examination as well as high serum IgG4 and IgG4/IgG ratio, although the serum markers are elevated in ~70% of patients. Guidelines for diagnosis of IgG4-related disease in general were proposed in 2011, revised in 2017.[45,46] According to the guidelines, (1) typical organ involvement, (2) serum IgG4 level, and (3) histopathological findings are used for diagnosis, where (1) + (2) + (3) indicates definite, (1) + (2) indicates possible, and (1) + (3) indicates probable. For intracranial cases, Lindstrom and colleagues[47] first proposed application of the consensus criteria (≥10 IgG4-positive cells/HPF as minimum criteria for the diagnosis). Leporati proposed specific criteria for the diagnosis of IgG4-RD hypophysitis.[48]

	Criterion	Diagnosis
1	Mononuclear infiltration of the pituitary gland, rich in lymphocytes and plasma cells, with >10 IgG4-positive cells/high-power field	Criterion 1 Or Criteria 2 + 3 Or Criteria 2 + 4 + 5
2	Sellar mass or thickened pituitary stalk by MRI	
3	Biopsy-proven involvement in other organs	
4	Serum IgG4 level >140 mg/dL (1.4 g/L)	
5	Shrinkage of the pituitary mass and symptom improvement with corticosteroids	

PROGNOSIS

Spontaneous improvement is very rare, and most of the cases show slow and indolent progression. IgG4-RD should be promptly treated with glucocorticoids, which often cause remission within a few weeks. However, long-term maintenance glucocorticoid therapy, with or without a steroid-sparing agent, may be required. Relapse is possible and multiple courses of high-dose glucocorticoids are often necessary. Rituximab and azathioprine have also been reported to be effective.

Pathologic Key Features— IgG4-Related Disease

An autoimmune disease that may affect other organs, IgG4-related disease is manifest in the sellar region as hypopituitarism, diabetes insipidus, or mass effect

May present as a pachymeningitis or hypophysitis

Diagnosis requires a combination of histopathologic, radiologic, and serologic criteria

Histopathologic features include more than 10 IgG4-positive cells/high-power field within a lymphoplasmacytic infiltrate, storiform fibrosis, and obliterative phlebitis

RATHKE CLEFT CYST

INTRODUCTION

Rathke Cleft Cysts (RC) are benign, epithelium-lined intrasellar cysts that originate from remnants of the Rathke pouch. They are found in 13% to 33% of the general population and can compress adjacent structures, causing symptoms such as headaches, vision problems, or pituitary hormone deficits.

Most radiologically diagnosed RCs may be managed conservatively, because they are statistically unlikely to increase in size or cause symptoms.

However, among patients who present with sellar and suprasellar lesions in neurosurgical series, RCs account for 6% to 10%.

GROSS FEATURES

RCs commonly have a round, ovoid, or dumbbell shape on imaging studies, given their location between anterior and posterior gland. On computed tomography (CT) scan, they are well-circumscribed, hypoattenuating, cystic sellar masses that may extend into the suprasellar region.[49] Because of the variability of cyst contents, RCs are either isoattenuating or hyperattenuating relative to the brain

parenchyma. Typically, there is a thin wall that may enhance. Extravasation of cystic contents may also cause enhancement. Complex cysts may have septations. Large cysts may cause bone remodeling.

MRI appearances of RCs are highly variable but can be roughly categorized into 2 patterns: those with low intensity on T1-weighted and high intensity on T2-weighted images, and those with high intensity on T1-weighted images and variable intensity on T2-weighted images. Most are homogenous, as opposed to other lesions, such as craniopharyngioma, which are more heterogeneous. However, the features on standard sequences of cystic lesions (RC, craniopharyngioma, and hemorrhagic and cystic pituitary adenomas) often overlap. Data suggest that a RC may be differentiated from a craniopharyngioma or a hemorrhagic pituitary adenoma using special diffusion-weighted imaging techniques.[50]

MICROSCOPIC FEATURES

Given their location between anterior and posterior pituitary, the cyst wall may be adjacent to normal components of these structures. The lining ranges from low cuboidal to tall columnar, sometimes with mucinous differentiation (**Fig. 10**), consistently reactive for pan-cytokeratin. Cilia are present on high-power magnification. The lining may also undergo squamous metaplasia. RCs often contain colloid-like, eosinophilic, amorphous mucin.

DIFFERENTIAL DIAGNOSIS

Squamous metaplasia may be confused for papillary craniopharyngioma in a small biopsy; BRAF V600E immunohistochemistry may help to distinguish the two. An epidermoid cyst may be considered, although the presence of a keratohyaline layer and flaky keratin content will distinguish it from RC.

DIAGNOSIS

Neuroimaging studies alone, given the variability in presentation, are often insufficient to make a definitive diagnosis. The neuroimaging differential includes arachnoid cyst, epidermoid cyst, craniopharyngioma, or pituitary adenoma. Tissue diagnosis remains a gold standard.

PROGNOSIS

The outcome of a symptomatic RC is related to anterior pituitary dysfunction, central diabetes insipidus, visual deficits, and other symptoms related to mass effect, and possibly the granulomatous, xanthomatous, and lymphocytic

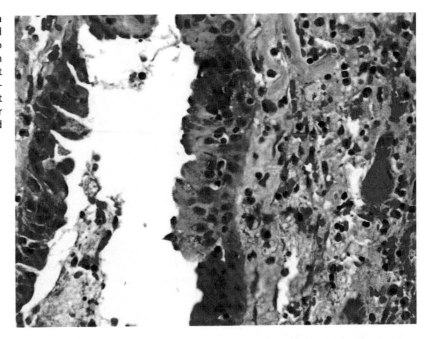

Fig. 10. Presence of a cyst lining with ciliated low cuboidal to columnar epithelium with or without mucinous cells characterizes Rathke Cleft Cyst (RC). This particular example shows scattered intracytoplasmic mucin.

hypophysitis theorized to occur after rupture of RC.[51–53] Symptoms resolve in most of the patients following surgical resection, although diabetes insipidus may persist.[54]

Pathologic Key Features
– RATHKE CLEFT CYST

Simple or complex cyst arising from the Rathke cleft remnant lined by cuboidal, columnar, or attenuated respiratory epithelium may undergo squamous metaplasia and contains eosinophilic- or colloid-like contents.

CRANIOPHARYNGIOMA

INTRODUCTION

Craniopharyngiomas are WHO grade I, circumscribed epithelial tumors that most commonly arise in the suprasellar region. Craniopharyngioma comprises 5% to 10% of all childhood brain tumors and 1.2% to 4.6% of brain tumors in adults.[3] The peak incidence is in children aged 0 to 19 years. A second peak occurs later in life, between ages 40 and 79 years. There is no sex predilection.

Craniopharyngioma comprises 2 clinically, histologically, and biologically distinct subtypes: adamantinomatous (most common) and papillary. Rare hybrid forms have also been reported, even with the characteristic genetic signatures (see later discussion).[55] Papillary craniopharyngioma occurs almost exclusively in adults, whereas adamantinomatous craniopharyngioma occurs in both adults and children.

The close histopathologic and immunohistochemical resemblance among adamantinomatous craniopharyngioma, adamantinoma of the jaw, and calcifying odontogenic cyst suggests an odontogenic epithelial differentiation for these tumors.[56] Collision lesions of craniopharyngioma with, most commonly, pituitary adenoma, have been described.[57,58]

The current hypothesis is that pituitary adenoma, adamantinomatous craniopharyngioma, and Rathke cyst share a common ancestry from involuted remnants of the Rathke pouch and the craniopharyngeal duct.[59] In elderly persons, squamous metaplasia of adenohypophyseal cells of the pituitary stalk or gland has been postulated as a possible origin for the papillary variant of craniopharyngioma.[60]

Clinical features of craniopharyngiomas may include visual disturbances (from compression of the optic chiasm and adjacent nerves and tracts), endocrine abnormalities, including diabetes insipidus, and signs of increased intracranial pressure. Cognitive and personality changes have also been observed.

GROSS FEATURES

MRI typically shows an adamantinomatous craniopharyngioma as a complex solid/cystic lesion with

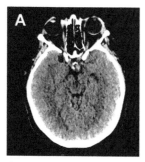
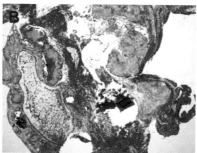
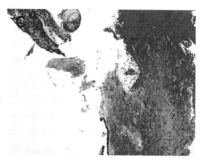

Fig. 11. Peripheral calcifications of adamantinomatous craniopharyngioma are a helpful feature in their diagnosis on CT scan (*A*). Wet keratin, peripheral palisading, stellate reticulum, and dystrophic calcifications are variably present on histologic examination (*B*). Piloid gliosis with numerous Rosenthal material is often seen at the periphery of adamantinomatous craniopharyngioma and can be a diagnostic pitfall during intraoperative consultation (*C*).

heterogeneous signal intensity. The cysts are often filled with fluid of high protein content and are hyperintense on T1-weighted images. Solid areas enhance. Peripheral calcification is often prominent on CT scans (**Fig. 11**A).

Adamantinomatous craniopharyngioma is a partly cystic mass filled with dark greenish-brown fluid that has traditionally been compared in terms of color and consistency with "machinery oil." The characteristic white speckled appearance of "wet" keratin nodules typical of the adamantinomatous variant is frequently seen on gross examination.

MRI of a papillary craniopharyngioma characteristically depicts an enhancing, predominantly solid, circumscribed mass without the calcification or complex cystic architecture of the adamantinomatous variant. The papillary architecture may sometimes be evident.

In contrast to the adamantinomatous variant, which tends to insinuate tongues around nerves and blood vessels, the papillary subtype is comparatively well circumscribed and typically lacks the complex multicystic architecture and fluid-filled spaces.

Although the imaging descriptions of the 2 morphologic variants are typically described as earlier, note that overlap and exceptions occur. In addition, there is overlap between the imaging characteristics of craniopharyngiomas of both subtypes and other sellar/suprasellar mass lesions of this anatomic neighborhood; thus, tissue examination is generally required for definitive diagnosis.

MICROSCOPIC FEATURES

With adamantinomatous craniopharyngiomas, a complex epithelial lesion with cysts and calcified "wet" keratin is seen. The epithelium has central stellate reticulum with prominent peripheral palisading. Rarely, ciliated cells and goblet cells are encountered. Even more rare is enamel formation in an abortive attempt to form "toothlike" structures (**Fig. 11**B). The adjacent neural parenchyma may show granulomatous reaction with cholesterol clefts. In some cases, there is perilesional piloid gliosis with Rosenthal fibers (**Fig. 11**C). A biopsy or frozen section sample from this area can be potentially misleading.

With papillary craniopharyngiomas, an epithelial lesion composed of mature squamous epithelium without surface maturation, a keratohyaline granular layer, or keratin formation is noted (**Fig. 12**A). Focal tissue dehiscence with resultant pseudopapillary architecture is often present, as are small whorls. Although basal peripheral palisading is also seen, this feature is not as prominent as with the adamantinomatous variant. The most characteristic features of the adamantinomatous subtype are absent, including nodules of "wet" keratin, "stellate reticulum," and calcification. Rarely, ciliated epithelium and goblet cells may be encountered. Immunostain for BRAF (V600E) tends to be positive (**Fig. 12**B).

DIFFERENTIAL DIAGNOSIS

The histopathologic differential includes epidermoid cyst, possibly germinoma, Rathke cleft cyst with squamous metaplasia, and pilocytic astrocytoma (in areas of surrounding piloid gliosis) in small biopsy samples.

DIAGNOSIS

Craniopharyngioma tumor cells display immunoreactivity to epithelial membrane antigen (EMA) and cytokeratin. Most adamantinomatous craniopharyngiomas show aberrant nuclear expression of beta-catenin, a feature that is not typically observed in papillary craniopharyngiomas.[61] In contrast, most papillary craniopharyngiomas harbor BRAF V600E mutation, which can be demonstrated immunohistochemically.[62]

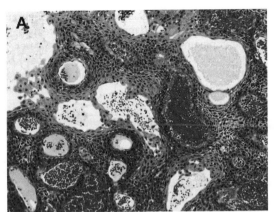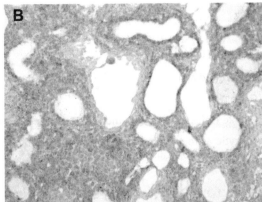

Fig. 12. Papillary craniopharyngioma. Well-differentiated stratified squamous epithelium with pseudopapillary architecture and lacking keratohyaline granules with pseudopapillary architecture (*A*). Reactivity with BRAF (V600E) immunostain is a frequent finding and can help distinguish with its close mimics such as epidermoid cyst (*B*).

PROGNOSIS

Craniopharyngioma is managed by 1 of 2 strategies: (1) attempted gross total resection or (2) a planned subtotal resection followed by radiotherapy or other adjuvant therapy. No established guidelines exist regarding management of craniopharyngioma. Radiation therapy includes external fractionated radiation, stereotactic radiation, or brachytherapy. In addition, bleomycin may be considered for local intracystic chemotherapy, particularly in children.[63]

Neuropsychological deficits represent the major limiting factor for independent social functioning. The degree of psychosocial impairment correlates directly with the degree of hypothalamic injury sustained at the time of surgery. In some patients, deficits are related to radiation injury.

Panhypopituitarism is reported in most of the patients. Most patients require multiple hormonal supplements and adjustments during long-term follow-up. Other prevalent morbidities include neurologic, psychosocial, and cardiovascular abnormalities.

OVERVIEW: MOLECULAR PATHOLOGY OF CRANIOPHARYNGIOMA

Most of the adamantinomatous craniopharyngiomas harbor a mutation of the beta-catenin gene (*CTNNB1*). Almost all mutations involve exon 3, which encodes the degradation targeting box of beta-catenin. This mutation results in nuclear accumulation of beta-catenin protein and dysregulation of the Wnt signaling pathway, with activation of downstream targets such as Axin-2. Papillary craniopharyngiomas and other sellar region lesions do not exhibit this mutation.

BRAF V600E mutations have been demonstrated in up to 95% of papillary craniopharyngioma cases.[32] This is a well-studied activating mutation of a serine-threonine kinase involved in cell division and differentiation via the MAP-kinase/ERK signaling pathway, which has been implicated in a variety of other neoplasms including melanoma, colorectal carcinoma, and papillary thyroid carcinoma.

A study reported 2 cases of adamantinomatous craniopharyngioma exhibiting *BRAF V600E* mutations; however, in both cases a concomitant *CTNNB1* mutation was also present.[55] In most cases, however, BRAF V600E and beta-catenin alterations segregate by subtype.

ASSOCIATED GENETIC CHANGES/ALTERATIONS

Relatively recent studies have also demonstrated that papillary and adamantinomatous craniopharyngiomas have distinct DNA methylation profiles.[64] Chromosomal imbalances are very rare in both subtypes.[65,66]

 Pathologic Key Features—Craniopharyngioma

Two types: adamantinomatous (adults and children, *CTNNB1* mutations), and papillary (adults, *BRAFV600E* mutations)

Adamantinomatous variant: a complex epithelial lesion with cysts and calcified "wet" keratin; central stellate reticulum with prominent peripheral palisading

Papillary variant: epithelial lesion composed of mature squamous epithelium without surface maturation, a keratohyaline granular layer, or keratin formation; focal tissue dehiscence results in pseudopapillary architecture

Adjacent piloid gliosis may be a diagnostic pitfall

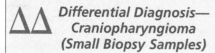

**Differential Diagnosis—
Craniopharyngioma
(Small Biopsy Samples)**

Epidermoid cyst

Germinoma

Rathke cleft cyst with squamous metaplasia

Pilocytic astrocytoma or other low-grade glial neoplasm (piloid gliosis)

PITUICYTOMA, SPINDLE CELL ONCOCYTOMA, AND GRANULAR CELL TUMOR OF NEUROHYPOPHYSIS

INTRODUCTION

These 3 WHO grade I tumors are derivatives of posterior gland pituicytes, and as such, are TTF-1 immunoreactive. Overall, they are rare, and may present incidentally, at autopsy or in association with other endocrine neoplasms or hemorrhage. Granular cell tumor (GCT) most commonly is noted as an incidental finding.

GROSS FEATURES

Neuroimaging features are similar to pituitary adenoma.

MICROSCOPIC FEATURES

Pituitcytoma is a spindle cell neoplasm, with plump cells in a fascicular architecture (**Fig. 13**). Mitoses are rare. Considered a mitochondria-rich

variant of pituicytoma, spindle cell oncocytoma shows more epithelioid morphology, more evident nuclear pleomorphism (**Fig. 14**), and at times a lymphocytic infiltrate. Similarly, GCT may be considered as a lysosomal-rich variant of pituicytoma and resembles GCT in other anatomic locations.

DIFFERENTIAL DIAGNOSIS

Meningioma may seem similar to pituicytoma, but the latter lacks characteristic features such as whorls and calcification.

DIAGNOSIS

Pituicytoma is positive for S100 and TTF-1, with variable reactivity for GFAP.

PROGNOSIS

Surgery is the only curative option; recurrence and complications are common.[67]

**Pathologic Key Features—
Tumors of the Posterior
Pituitary**

TTF1-positive tumors considered to be related by cell of origin (posterior pituicytes)

Pituicytoma: spindle cells

Spindle cell oncocytoma: mitochondrial-rich variant; more epithelioid morphology

Granular cell tumor: lysosomal-rich variant; similar to GCT in other locations

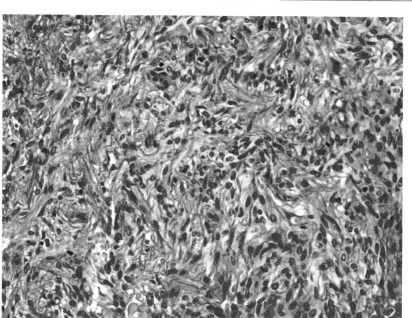

Fig. 13. Pituicytoma with spindled cells arranged in a fascicular arrangement with paucity of mitotic activity and pleomorphism.

METASTASES

INTRODUCTION

Although metastases to the pituitary (MP) are overall rare (~1% in surgical series of transsphenoidal surgery for sellar lesions, ~5% in autopsy for systemic cancers, and 17% in autopsy for breast cancer in particular), rates are increasing, presumably due to improved patient survival.[68] Breast and lung carcinomas are the most common malignancies to metastasize to the sellar region. Almost always, MP are part of widespread metastases, involving at least 5 other sites (often osseous), affecting patients in the sixth to seventh decades. Occasionally, MP are the first presentation of an occult tumor, and they can also occur in young adulthood.

Clinically, MP most often present with diabetes insipidus, reflecting a predilection to involve the posterior pituitary.[68] Anterior pituitary and cranial nerve deficits may occur as well, however. Hyperprolactinemia resulting from "stalk effect" has also been described.

GROSS FEATURES

When radiographically detectable, MP show similar features to primary sellar tumors, particularly pituitary adenoma.[68]

MICROSCOPIC FEATURES

Metastatic malignancies will reflect their primary origin but on small, crushed samples, can be difficult to distinguish from a primary sellar tumor.

DIFFERENTIAL DIAGNOSIS

The differential diagnosis often depends on the morphologic appearance of the primary, but pituitary adenoma can often enter the differential of a metastatic tumor.

DIAGNOSIS

Diagnosis is based on a combination of clinical, radiologic, histomorphologic, and immunohistochemical features, perhaps with ancillary molecular or cytogenetic testing. Preoperative diagnosis of MP is difficult. CSF cytology from lumbar puncture may be useful when meningeal spread is present. The consideration of metastasis is crucial when evaluating a patient with a sellar tumor. The clinical presentation of diabetes insipidus can strongly suggest metastases over pituitary adenoma.[68]

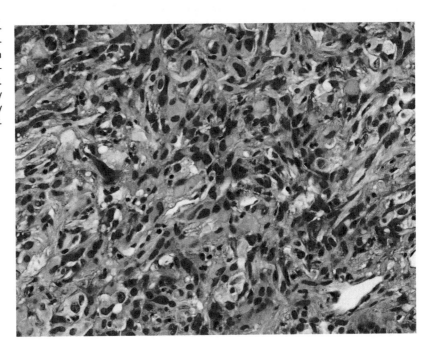

Fig. 14. Spindle cell oncocytoma with epithelioid to spindled cells in a vague fascicular architecture. Note the atypia. However, it is generally not accompanied by increased mitotic activity.

PROGNOSIS

Prognosis will depend on the treatment of the primary, metastatic burden, and patient comorbidities.

SCHWANNOMA

INTRODUCTION

Schwannomas mostly originate from peripheral, often sensory nerves such as vestibular or trigeminal and account for 8% to 10% of all primary intracranial tumors. They are uncommon in the sellar region. The origin of primary schwannomas in the sellar region is still unclear. As the sellar region has no obvious nerve, it has been hypothesized that tumors originate from lateral sellar nerve plexus, perivascular schwann cells adjacent to the medial wall of the pituitary fossa, or sensory nerves of the dura.[69] Less than 30 cases of intrasellar schwannoma have been reported in the literature.[70] The clinical presentation is related to mass effect and compression of adjacent structures. Symptoms are similar to those caused by pituitary adenomas. Suprasellar expansion may cause visual disturbances.

GROSS FEATURES

As other sellar and suprasellar lesions, MRI is the modality of choice for imaging schwannomas. However, the imaging features overlap with pituitary adenoma. On T1-weighted sequences, schwannoma is isointense or hypointense compared with gray matter and shows homogeneous enhancement with contrast. On T2-weighted images, schwannomas are more likely hyperintense than pituitary adenoma. Diffusion-weighted imaging and apparent diffusion coefficient maps show higher values with firm or fibrous tumors. Computed tomography may help show bony destruction and bony anatomy relevant for surgical planning.

Generally, schwannomas are circumscribed and may show a pseudocapsule. In the sellar region, almost all of reported tumors are firm and hypervascular.[71]

MICROSCOPIC FEATURES

Histologically, schwannomas are spindle-cell neoplasms with relatively minimal pleomorphism. Hyper- and hypocellular areas (Antoni A and B, respectively) and Verocay bodies are characteristic features. Occasional profound nuclear enlargement and atypia may be seen ("degenerative" or "ancient" change). Thick-walled blood vessels are also common.

DIFFERENTIAL DIAGNOSIS

Other spindle cell neoplasms may mimic schwannoma, including fibrous meningioma and pituicytoma. Schwannomas typically show intense reaction with S-100, collagen IV, and vimentin but are negative for EMA and glial fibrillary acidic protein (GFAP). In contrast, fibroblastic meningiomas are only moderately reactive to S-100, and pituicytomas are immunopositive for GFAP.

DIAGNOSIS

Diagnosis is made on histologic, immunohistochemical features in combination with the appropriate imaging and clinical scenarios.

PROGNOSIS

Schwannoma is a WHO grade I tumor, with surgical resection as the recommended treatment strategy.

> ### Pathologic Key Features—Schwannoma
>
> Spindle cell neoplasm with hyper and hypocellular areas, degenerative nuclear atypia, thick-walled blood vessels
>
> Diffusely S100-positive; collagen IV highlights basement membrane element
>
> Firm, hypervascular tumors

CHORDOMA

INTRODUCTION

Chordoma is a rare neoplasm considered to be of low to intermediate malignancy. It originates from notochord remnants and almost always occurs in a midline location. They are rare, representing less than 0.1% of all skull base tumors.[72] Among all chordomas, ~25% to 36% of the tumors are found in the skull base.[73] Strictly intrasellar chordomas are rare; sellar invasion is associated with clival tumors.[74]

GROSS FEATURES

By MRI, chordomas are usually hypointense on T1-weighted and hyperintense on T2-weighted images. There is a moderate to marked contrast enhancement. Because chordomas have lower

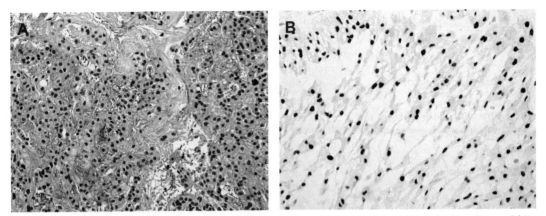

Fig. 15. Chordoma with tumor cells displaying only modest atypia, arranged in a "chordoid" pattern within a background of myxoid stroma (*A*). Physaliferous cells (multivacuolated "bubbly" cytoplasm) are seen often, albeit variably, present and are characteristic. Brachyury expression conforms to its notochordal lineage and is a consistent finding (*B*; diffuse nuclear positivity).

apparent diffusion coefficient (ADC) values, ADC can be useful to differentiate chordoma from chondrosarcoma.[75] On noncontrast CT, chordoma typically appears as well-circumscribed, hypoattenuating, heterogeneous lesion with extensive lytic bone destruction.[76]

Grossly, the tumor is a lobulated mass with a gelatinous or chondroid cut surface. When centered in bone, the tumor typically extends beyond the cortex into the surrounding soft tissue.[77]

MICROSCOPIC FEATURES

By definition, chordoma is a malignant (notochordal) tumor. The 2013 WHO classification splits chordomas into well-differentiated (classical myxoid, chondroid or mixed types) and dedifferentiated variants. The characteristic feature is vacuolated physaliferous cells, surrounded by a myxoid matrix, and arranged in a "chordoid pattern" (**Fig. 15**A). Brachyury expression (**Fig. 15**B), as well as lack of *IDH* 1 or 2 mutations, helps differentiate chordoma from chondrosarcoma.[78]

DIFFERENTIAL DIAGNOSIS

In the sellar region, the differential includes chondrosarcoma, metastatic carcinoma, and possibly, myoepithelial tumors extending from a head and neck primary.

DIAGNOSIS

A combination of imaging and microscopic features, as well as demonstration of brachyury expression, is diagnostic of chordoma.

PROGNOSIS

Chordoma is known to have aggressive local behavior and a high rate of recurrence. Metastasis may also occur; its long-term prognosis is poor. Resection using an endonasal endoscopic approach is recommended for skull base chordomas. However, because of their location and extension, radical resection is not always achievable. In addition, although an aggressive or radical resection approach has been suggested to be likely the most important factor influencing chordoma relapse and long-term patient survival, there is still no agreement on the standardized classification for the extent of tumor excision.[79] Proton beam therapy is increasingly recommended for chordomas.[80] Medical therapy options for recurrence include imatinib and sorafenib as palliative treatment options to slow disease progression or alleviate symptoms. In addition, several case reports have noted activity of sunitinib and epidermal growth factor receptor inhibitors (cetuximab, erlotinib, gefitinib).

Pathologic Key Features— Chordoma

Pathognomonic feature is the presence of physaliferous cells and attempts to form the notochord; positive for the transcription factor brachyury

WHO 2013 classification specifies well-differentiated (classical myxoid, chondroid or mixed types) and dedifferentiated variants

Differential Diagnosis— Chordoma

Low-grade chondrosarcoma

Metastatic carcinoma or myoepithelial neoplasm with direct extension from head and neck primary

Chondroma

Metaplastic meningioma

ATYPICAL TERATOID/RHABDOID TUMORS IN ADULTS

INTRODUCTION

Atypical teratoid/rhabdoid tumor (AT/RT), an embryonal, primary central nervous system (CNS) malignancy defined by the 2016 WHO by loss of INI1 (alterations in *SMARCB1* gene) or BRG1 (alterations in *SMARC4A* gene) protein expression and often composed partly by "rhabdoid" cells, most commonly occurs in children younger than 3 years. However, several cases have now been described in adults, both in the sellar region (~46% of 50 cases identified in adults) and elsewhere in the neuraxis.[81]

GROSS FEATURES

On MRI, AT/RTs are isodense to hyperintense on FLAIR images and show restricted diffusion. Most tumors are variably contrast enhancing. Leptomeningeal dissemination at presentation is less commonly reported in adults (4%) as opposed to the pediatric population (~25%). Grossly, the tissue is similar to medulloblastoma and is soft, pinkish-red, demarcated from adjacent parenchyma, and necrotic with hemorrhage.

MICROSCOPIC FEATURES

AT/RTs are variegated, primitive-appearing tumors. The definitive feature is a population of rhabdoid cells, characterized by eccentric nuclei containing vesicular chromatin, prominent eosinophilic nucleoli, abundant cytoplasm, and eosinophilic globular cytoplasmic inclusions. Usually, this is a minor population. Other components of the tumor include primitive neuroectodermal, mesenchymal, and epithelial, with the small-cell neuroectodermal component being most frequent among these.

DIFFERENTIAL DIAGNOSIS

The differential diagnosis includes any primitive-appearing malignancy, including metastases.

DIAGNOSIS

Diagnosis is based on the loss of INI1 or BRG1 proteins by immunohistochemistry or by demonstration of alterations in *SMARCB1* or *SMARC4A* genes. Other immunostains may be useful, including EMA, SMA, and vimentin in rhabdoid cells; GFAP, neurofilament protein, and synaptophysin are also commonly expressed. Germ cell markers and skeletal muscle markers are not typically expressed.

PROGNOSIS

Given the limited number of AT/RT cases in adults, overall prognosis and impact of extent of resection and adjuvant therapy remains unclear. Of 50 patients, 31 (62%) died, with an average time to death of 20 months (0–168 months). Of 28 patients who received combined radiotherapy and chemotherapy, 15 were alive at follow-up, ranging from 6 months to 17 years. Time to death for the remaining 13 of these 28 ranged from 3 months to 3 years after diagnosis. There was no statistically significant difference in outcome for patients with and without gross total resection.[81]

Pathologic Key Features— Atypical Teratoid/Rhabdoid Tumor in Adults

Primitive, high-grade malignancy rarely found in adults

Alterations of the *SMARCB1* or *SMARC4A* genes (loss of INI1 or BRG1 protein respectively)

Rhabdoid cells are a rare but defining feature

Primitive neuroectodermal (predominant), mesenchymal, and epithelial components

Differential Diagnosis— Atypical Teratoid/ Rhabdoid Tumor in Adults

Metastatic poorly differentiated malignancy

Malignant germ cell tumor

High-grade lymphoma

Other high-grade primary CNS neoplasm with embryonal features

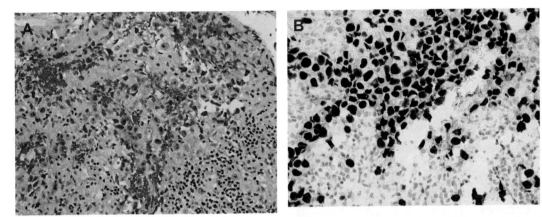

Fig. 16. Germinoma. As elsewhere, germinoma is composed of dual cell population. Although the neoplastic cells are large with pale eosinophilic to vacuolated cytoplasm with vesicular nuclei and prominent nucleoli, the intermixed lymphocytes are nonneoplastic (*A*). Sometimes they can be associated with significant granulomatous inflammation, which can be a diagnostic pitfall on small biopsies. Diffuse and strong nuclear expression of OCT3/4 within tumor cells is diagnostic (*B*).

OTHER TUMORS MAY OCCUR IN THE SELLAR REGION

As a final note, other tumors may present in the sellar region, including germ cell tumors (**Fig. 16**), diffuse midline glioma defined by H3 K27M mutation, optic pathway glioma, chondrosarcoma, lipoma, meningioma, paraganglioma, gangliocytoma, hemangioblastoma, solitary fibrous tumor/hemangiopericytoma, hematopoietic neoplasms including Langerhans cell histiocytosis (**Fig. 17**) as well as plasma cell neoplasms, melanomas, and metastases have

all been described. The histopathologic features of these tumors are characteristic and not unique to this location. Local extension from a nasal, sinonasal, or nasopharyngeal malignancy is also not infrequent (**Fig. 18**).

DISCLOSURE

The authors have no relevant financial or commercial disclosures. No specific funding sources were used in the writing of this article.

Fig. 17. Langerhan cell histiocytosis with sheets of histiocytic cells containing nuclear groves and scattered multinucleate giant cells harboring similar nuclear features. Eosinophils may not always be prominent and can be only focally present or lacking. Strong immunoreactivity with CD1a is a consistent feature.

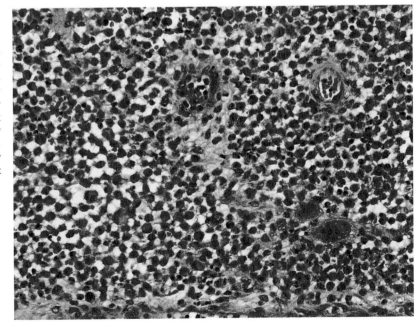

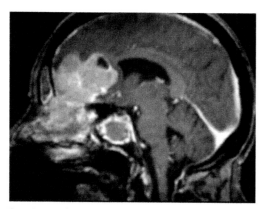

Fig. 18. Local invasion from a surrounding nasal/paranasal malignancy is not uncommon. MRI from a patient with olfactory neuroblastoma demonstrating marked intracranial extension with involvement of the sella and brain.

REFERENCES

1. Chen J, Schmidt RE, Dahiya S. Pituitary adenoma in pediatric and adolescent populations. J Neuropathol Exp Neurol 2019. https://doi.org/10.1093/jnen/nlz040.
2. Ostrom QT, Gittleman H, Truitt G, et al. CBTRUS statistical report: primary brain and other central nervous system tumors diagnosed in the United States in 2011-2015. Neuro Oncol 2018. https://doi.org/10.1093/neuonc/noy131.
3. Ostrom QT, Gittleman H, Liao P, et al. CBTRUS statistical report: primary brain and other central nervous system tumors diagnosed in the United States in 2010-2014. Neuro Oncol 2017. https://doi.org/10.1093/neuonc/nox158.
4. Lopes MBS. The 2017 World Health Organization classification of tumors of the pituitary gland: a summary. Acta Neuropathol 2017. https://doi.org/10.1007/s00401-017-1769-8.
5. Al-Shraim M, Asa SL. The 2004 World Health Organization classification of pituitary tumors: what is new? Acta Neuropathol 2006. https://doi.org/10.1007/s00401-005-1093-6.
6. Zaidi HA, Cote DJ, Dunn IF, et al. Predictors of aggressive clinical phenotype among immunohistochemically confirmed atypical adenomas. J Clin Neurosci 2016. https://doi.org/10.1016/j.jocn.2016.09.014.
7. Trouillas J, Roy P, Sturm N, et al. A new prognostic clinicopathological classification of pituitary adenomas: a multicentric case-control study of 410 patients with 8 years post-operative follow-up. Acta Neuropathol 2013. https://doi.org/10.1007/s00401-013-1084-y.
8. Miermeister CP, Petersenn S, Buchfelder M, et al. Histological criteria for atypical pituitary adenomas - data from the German pituitary adenoma registry suggests modifications. Acta Neuropathol Commun 2015. https://doi.org/10.1186/s40478-015-0229-8.
9. Chiloiro S, Doglietto F, Trapasso B, et al. Typical and atypical pituitary adenomas: a single-center analysis of outcome and prognosis. Neuroendocrinology 2015. https://doi.org/10.1159/000375448.
10. Bonneville JF. Magnetic resonance imaging of pituitary tumors. Front Horm Res 2016. https://doi.org/10.1159/000442327.
11. Hardy J, Vezina JL. Transsphenoidal neurosurgery of intracranial neoplasm. Adv Neurol 1976;15:261-73.
12. Knosp E, Steiner E, Kitz K, et al. Pituitary adenomas with invasion of the cavernous sinus space: a magnetic resonance imaging classification compared with surgical findings. Neurosurgery 1993. https://doi.org/10.1227/00006123-199310000-00008.
13. Gonçalves MB, De Oliveira JG, Williams HA, et al. Cavernous sinus medial wall: dural or fibrous layer? Systematic review of the literature. Neurosurg Rev 2012. https://doi.org/10.1007/s10143-011-0360-3.
14. Frank G, Pasquini E. Endoscopic endonasal cavernous sinus surgery, with special reference to pituitary adenomas. Front Horm Res 2006. https://doi.org/10.1159/000091573.
15. Bao X, Deng K, Liu X, et al. Extended transsphenoidal approach for pituitary adenomas invading the cavernous sinus using multiple complementary techniques. Pituitary 2016. https://doi.org/10.1007/s11102-015-0675-0.
16. Woodworth GF, Patel KS, Shin B, et al. Surgical outcomes using a medial-to-lateral endonasal endoscopic approach to pituitary adenomas invading the cavernous sinus: clinical article. J Neurosurg 2014. https://doi.org/10.3171/2014.1.JNS131228.
17. Dhandapani S, Singh H, Negm HM, et al. Cavernous sinus invasion in pituitary adenomas: systematic review and pooled data meta-analysis of radiologic criteria and comparison of endoscopic and microscopic surgery. World Neurosurg 2016. https://doi.org/10.1016/j.wneu.2016.08.088.
18. McDonald WC, Banerji N, McDonald KN, et al. Steroidogenic factor 1, pit-1, and adrenocorticotropic hormone: a rational starting place for the immunohistochemical characterization of pituitary adenoma. Arch Pathol Lab Med 2017. https://doi.org/10.5858/arpa.2016-0082-OA.
19. Lloyd RV, Osamura RY, Klöppel G, et al. Pathology and genetics of tumours of endocrine organs. 4th edition. Lyon, France: WHO; 2017.
20. Obari A, Sano T, Ohyama K, et al. Clinicopathological features of growth hormone-producing pituitary adenomas: difference among various types defined by cytokeratin distribution pattern including a transitional form. Endocr Pathol 2008. https://doi.org/10.1007/s12022-008-9029-z.

21. Cuevas-Ramos D, Carmichael JD, Cooper O, et al. A structural and functional acromegaly classification. J Clin Endocrinol Metab 2015. https://doi.org/10.1210/jc.2014-2468.

22. Kreutzer J, Vance ML, Lopes MBS, et al. Surgical management of GH-secreting pituitary adenomas: an outcome study using modern remission criteria. J Clin Endocrinol Metab 2001. https://doi.org/10.1210/jcem.86.9.7819.

23. Saeger W, Ludecke DK, Buchfelder M, et al. Pathohistological classification of pituitary tumors: 10 years of experience with the German Pituitary Tumor Registry. Eur J Endocrinol 2007;156(2):203–16.

24. Kontogeorgos G, Horvath E, Kovacs K, et al. Morphologic changes of prolactin-producing pituitary adenomas after short treatment with dopamine agonists. Acta Neuropathol 2006. https://doi.org/10.1007/s00401-005-1111-8.

25. Hamester U, Saeger W, Ludecke DK. Light microscopical morphometry of prolactin secreting adenomas under treatment with dopamine agonists. Histol Histopathol 1987;2(2):135–42.

26. Mete O, Cintosun A, Pressman I, et al. Epidemiology and biomarker profile of pituitary adenohypophysial tumors. Mod Pathol 2018. https://doi.org/10.1038/s41379-018-0016-8.

27. Clarke MJ, Erickson D, Castro MR, et al. Thyroid-stimulating hormone pituitary adenomas. J Neurosurg 2008. https://doi.org/10.3171/JNS/2008/109/7/0017.

28. Mete O, Gomez-Hernandez K, Kucharczyk W, et al. Silent subtype 3 pituitary adenomas are not always silent and represent poorly differentiated monomorphous plurihormonal Pit-1 lineage adenomas. Mod Pathol 2016. https://doi.org/10.1038/modpathol.2015.151.

29. Lopes MBS, Sloan E, Polder J. Mixed gangliocytoma-pituitary adenoma. Insights on the pathogenesis of a rare sellar tumor. Am J Surg Pathol 2017. https://doi.org/10.1097/PAS.0000000000000806.

30. Jiang X, Zhang X. The molecular pathogenesis of pituitary adenomas: an update. Endocrinol Metab (Seoul) 2013. https://doi.org/10.3803/enm.2013.28.4.245.

31. Faltermeier CM, Magill ST, Blevins L, et al. Molecular biology of pituitary adenomas. Neurosurg Clin N Am 2019. https://doi.org/10.1016/j.nec.2019.05.001.

32. Bi WL, Larsen AG, Dunn IF. Genomic alterations in sporadic pituitary tumors. Curr Neurol Neurosci Rep 2018. https://doi.org/10.1007/s11910-018-0811-0.

33. Rostomyan L, Daly AF, Petrossians P, et al. Clinical and genetic characterization of pituitary gigantism: an international collaborative study in 208 patients. Endocr Relat Cancer 2015. https://doi.org/10.1530/ERC-15-0320.

34. Rostomyan L, Potorac I, Beckers P, et al. AIP mutations and gigantism. Ann Endocrinol (Paris) 2017. https://doi.org/10.1016/j.ando.2017.04.012.

35. Roohi J. Gigantism, acromegaly, and GPR101 mutations. N Engl J Med 2015. https://doi.org/10.1056/NEJMc1500340#SA2.

36. Doros L, Schultz KA, Stewart DR, et al. DICER1-related disorders. In: Adam MP, Ardinger HH, Pagon RA, et al, editors. GeneReviews® [Internet]. Seattle (WA): University of Washington; 2014.

37. Joshi MN, Whitelaw BC, Palomar MTP, et al. Immune checkpoint inhibitor-related hypophysitis and endocrine dysfunction: clinical review. Clin Endocrinol (Oxf) 2016. https://doi.org/10.1111/cen.13063.

38. Angelousi A, Chatzellis E, Kaltsas G. New molecular, biological, and immunological agents inducing hypophysitis. Neuroendocrinology 2017. https://doi.org/10.1159/000480086.

39. Ramos-Leví AM, Gargallo M, Serrano-Somavilla A, et al. Hypophysitis following treatment with Ustekinumab: radiological and pathological findings. Front Endocrinol (Lausanne) 2018. https://doi.org/10.3389/fendo.2018.00083. Available at:http://sfxit.ugent.be/ugent?sid=EMBASE&issn=16642392&id=doi:10.3389%2Ffendo.2018.00083&atitle=Hypophysitis+following+treatment+with+Ustekinumab%3A+Radiological+and+pathological+findings&stitle=Front.+Endocrinol.&title=Frontiers+in+Endocrinology&volume=9&issue=MAR&spage=&epage=&aulast=Ramos-Lev%C3%AD&aufirst=Ana+M.&auinit=A.M.&aufull=Ramos-Lev%C3%AD+A.M.&coden=&isbn=&pages=-&date=2018&auinit1=A&auinitm=M.

40. Karaca Z, Kelestimur F. The management of hypophysitis. Minerva Endocrinol 2016;41(3):390–9.

41. Joshi MN, Whitelaw BC, Carroll PV. Hypophysitis: diagnosis and treatment. Eur J Endocrinol 2018. https://doi.org/10.1530/EJE-17-0009.

42. Pekic S, Bogosavljevic V, Peker S, et al. Lymphocytic hypophysitis successfully treated with stereotactic radiosurgery: case report and review of the literature. J Neurol Surg A Cent Eur Neurosurg 2018. https://doi.org/10.1055/s-0037-1604079.

43. Shikuma J, Kan K, Ito R, et al. Critical review of IgG4-related hypophysitis. Pituitary 2017. https://doi.org/10.1007/s11102-016-0773-7.

44. Yuen KCJ, Moloney KJ, Mercado JU, et al. A case series of atypical features of patients with biopsy-proven isolated IgG4-related hypophysitis and normal serum IgG4 levels. Pituitary 2018. https://doi.org/10.1007/s11102-017-0852-4.

45. Rheumatology M, Ky AS. Comprehensive diagnostic criteria for IgG4- related disease (IgG4-RD), 2011 comprehensive diagnostic criteria for IgG4-related disease. Mod Rheumatol 2012. https://doi.org/10.1007/s10165-011-0571-z.

46. Umehara H, Okazaki K, Nakamura T, et al. Current approach to the diagnosis of IgG4-related disease–Combination of comprehensive diagnostic and organ-specific criteria. Mod Rheumatol 2017. https://doi.org/10.1080/14397595.2017.1290911.

47. Lindstrom KM, Cousar JB, Lopes MBS. IgG4-related meningeal disease: clinico-pathological features and proposal for diagnostic criteria. Acta Neuropathol 2010. https://doi.org/10.1007/s00401-010-0746-2.

48. Leporati P, Landek-Salgado MA, Lupi I, et al. IgG4-related hypophysitis: a new addition to the hypophysitis spectrum. J Clin Endocrinol Metab 2011. https://doi.org/10.1210/jc.2010-2970.

49. Naylor MF, Scheithauer BW, Forbes GS, et al. Rathke cleft cyst: Ct, mr, and pathology of 23 cases. J Comput Assist Tomogr 1995. https://doi.org/10.1097/00004728-199511000-00003.

50. Kunii N, Abe T, Kawamo M, et al. Rathke's cleft cysts: differentiation from other cystic lesions in the pituitary fossa by use of single-shot fast spin-echo diffusion-weighted MR imaging. Acta Neurochir (Wien) 2007. https://doi.org/10.1007/s00701-007-1234-x.

51. Duan K, Asa SL, Winer D, et al. Xanthomatous hypophysitis is associated with ruptured Rathke's Cleft cyst. Endocr Pathol 2017. https://doi.org/10.1007/s12022-017-9471-x.

52. Schittenhelm J, Beschorner R, Psaras T, et al. Rathke's cleft cyst rupture as potential initial event of a secondary perifocal lymphocytic hypophysitis: proposal of an unusual pathogenetic event and review of the literature. Neurosurg Rev 2008. https://doi.org/10.1007/s10143-008-0120-1.

53. Yang C, Wu H, Bao X, et al. Lymphocytic hypophysitis secondary to ruptured Rathke Cleft cyst: case report and literature review. World Neurosurg 2018. https://doi.org/10.1016/j.wneu.2018.03.086.

54. Kleinschmidt-DeMasters BK, Lillehei KO, Stears JC. The pathologic, surgical, and MR spectrum of Rathke cleft cysts. Surg Neurol 1995. https://doi.org/10.1016/0090-3019(95)00144-1.

55. Larkin SJ, Preda V, Karavitaki N, et al. BRAF V600E mutations are characteristic for papillary craniopharyngioma and may coexist with CTNNB1-mutated adamantinomatous craniopharyngioma. Acta Neuropathol 2014. https://doi.org/10.1007/s00401-014-1270-6.

56. Gomes CC, de Sousa SF, Gomez RS. Craniopharyngiomas and odontogenic tumors mimic normal odontogenesis and share genetic mutations, histopathologic features, and molecular pathways activation. Oral Surg Oral Med Oral Pathol Oral Radiol 2019. https://doi.org/10.1016/j.oooo.2018.11.004.

57. Finzi G, Cerati M, Marando A, et al. Mixed pituitary adenoma/craniopharyngioma: clinical, morphological, immunohistochemical and ultrastructural study of a case, review of the literature, and pathogenetic and nosological considerations. Pituitary 2014. https://doi.org/10.1007/s11102-013-0465-5.

58. Snyder R, Fayed I, Dowlati E, et al. Pituitary adenoma and craniopharyngioma collision tumor: diagnostic, treatment considerations, and review of the literature. World Neurosurg 2019. https://doi.org/10.1016/j.wneu.2018.10.048.

59. Garrè ML, Cama A. Craniopharyngioma: modern concepts in pathogenesis and treatment. Curr Opin Pediatr 2007. https://doi.org/10.1097/MOP.0b013e3282495a22.

60. Sato K, Oka H, Utsuki S, et al. Ciliated craniopharyngioma may arise from Rathke cleft cyst. Clin Neuropathol 2006;25(1):25–8.

61. Sekine S, Shibata T, Kokubu A, et al. Craniopharyngiomas of adamantinomatous type harbor β-Catenin gene mutations. Am J Pathol 2002. https://doi.org/10.1016/S0002-9440(10)64477-X.

62. Brastianos PK, Taylor-Weiner A, Manley PE, et al. Exome sequencing identifies BRAF mutations in papillary craniopharyngiomas. Nat Genet 2014. https://doi.org/10.1038/ng.2868.

63. Zhang S, Fang Y, Cai BW, et al. Intracystic bleomycin for cystic craniopharyngiomas in children. CochraneDatabase Syst Rev 2016. https://doi.org/10.1002/14651858.CD008890.pub4.

64. Hölsken A, Sill M, Merkle J, et al. Adamantinomatous and papillary craniopharyngiomas are characterized by distinct epigenomic as well as mutational and transcriptomic profiles. Acta Neuropathol Commun 2016. https://doi.org/10.1186/s40478-016-0287-6.

65. Rickert CH, Paulus W. Lack of chromosomal imbalances in adamantinomatous and papillary craniopharyngiomas. J Neurol Neurosurg Psychiatry 2003. https://doi.org/10.1136/jnnp.74.2.260.

66. Yoshimoto M, de Toledo SRC, da Silva NS, et al. Comparative genomic hybridization analysis of pediatric adamantinomatous craniopharyngiomas and a review of the literature. J Neurosurg 2004;101(1 Suppl):85–90.

67. Guerrero-Pérez F, Marengo AP, Vidal N, et al. Primary tumors of the posterior pituitary: a systematic review. Rev Endocr Metab Disord 2019. https://doi.org/10.1007/s11154-019-09484-1.

68. Komninos J, Vlassopoulou V, Protopapa D, et al. Tumors metastatic to the pituitary gland: case report and literature review. J Clin Endocrinol Metab 2004. https://doi.org/10.1210/jc.2003-030395.

69. Perez MT, Farkas J, Padron S, et al. Intrasellar and parasellar cellular schwannoma. Ann Diagn Pathol 2004. https://doi.org/10.1016/j.anndiagpath.2004.03.006.

70. Kong X, Wu H, Ma W, et al. Schwannoma in sellar region mimics invasive pituitary macroadenoma:

literature review with one case report. Medicine (Baltimore) 2016. https://doi.org/10.1097/MD.0000000000002931.

71. Zhang J, Xu S, Liu Q, et al. Intrasellar and Suprasellar Schwannoma misdiagnosed as pituitary macroadenoma: a case report and review of the literature. World Neurosurg 2016. https://doi.org/10.1016/j.wneu.2016.08.128.

72. Tzortzidis F, Elahi F, Wright D, et al. Patient outcome at long-term follow-up after aggressive microsurgical resection of cranial base chordomas. Neurosurgery 2006. https://doi.org/10.1227/01.NEU.0000223441.51012.9D.

73. Chugh R, Tawbi H, Lucas DR, et al. Chordoma: the nonsarcoma primary bone tumor. Oncologist 2007. https://doi.org/10.1634/theoncologist.12-11-1344.

74. Bresson D, Herman P, Polivka M, et al. Sellar lesions/pathology. Otolaryngol Clin North Am 2016. https://doi.org/10.1016/j.otc.2015.09.004.

75. Yeom KW, Lober RM, Mobley BC, et al. Diffusion-weighted MRI: distinction of skull base chordoma from chondrosarcoma. AJNR Am J Neuroradiol 2013. https://doi.org/10.3174/ajnr.A3333.

76. Santegoeds RGC, Temel Y, Beckervordersandforth JC, et al. State-of-the-art imaging in human chordoma of the skull base. Curr Radiol Rep 2018. https://doi.org/10.1007/s40134-018-0275-7.

77. Wasserman JK, Gravel D, Purgina B. Chordoma of the head and neck: a review. HeadNeck Pathol 2018. https://doi.org/10.1007/s12105-017-0860-8.

78. Oakley GJ, Fuhrer K, Seethala RR. Brachyury, SOX-9, and podoplanin, new markers in the skull base chordoma vs chondrosarcoma differential: a tissue microarray-based comparative analysis. Mod Pathol 2008. https://doi.org/10.1038/modpathol.2008.144.

79. Zou MX, Lv GH, Zhang QS, et al. Prognostic factors in skull base chordoma: a systematic literature review and meta-analysis. World Neurosurg 2018. https://doi.org/10.1016/j.wneu.2017.10.010.

80. Hulou MM, Garcia CR, Slone SA, et al. Comprehensive review of cranial chordomas using national databases in the USA. Clin Oncol 2019. https://doi.org/10.1016/j.clon.2019.06.004.

81. Chan V, Marro A, Max Findlay J, et al. A systematic review of atypical teratoid rhabdoid tumor in adults. Front Oncol 2018. https://doi.org/10.3389/fonc.2018.00567.

Iatrogenic Neuropathology of Systemic Therapies

Matthew Torre, MD, Mel B. Feany, MD, PhD*

KEYWORDS

- Iatrogenic • Neuropathology • Neurotoxicity • CAR T cell
- Immune effector cell-associated neurotoxicity syndrome (ICANS)
- Chemotherapy-related cognitive impairment

Key points

- Chimeric antigen receptor (CAR) T-cell–associated neurotoxicity (immune effector cell–associated neurotoxicity syndrome, ICANS) is closely associated with cytokine release syndrome and might be mediated by elevated circulating cytokines, endothelial activation, and impaired function of the blood-brain barrier (BBB).

- Histologic features of severe ICANS are varied and nonspecific but include perivascular fluid extravasation, platelet microthrombi, hemorrhage, microinfarcts, clasmatodendrosis, gliosis, microglial activation, and inflammatory cell infiltrate of variable extent, distribution, and composition (including CAR T cells).

- Adverse effects of chemotherapy involving the central nervous system (CNS) include leukoencephalopathy and chemotherapy-related cognitive impairment (CRCI).

- The pathogenesis of chemotherapy-induced leukoencephalopathy may involve the direct cytotoxic effect of chemotherapeutic agents on CNS progenitor cells and oligodendrocytes, impaired self-renewal potential of oligodendrocyte precursors exposed to sublethal chemotherapy concentrations, and oxidative stress.

- The pathogenesis underlying CRCI is multifactorial and likely includes elevated proinflammatory cytokines, reactive oxygen species (ROS)/oxidative stress, DNA damage, BBB dysfunction, direct effects of chemotherapy on CNS cells, neuroinflammation, and dysmyelination.

ABSTRACT

Administration of systemic antineoplastic agents can result in adverse neurologic events. We describe the clinicopathologic features and putative mechanisms underlying iatrogenic neuropathology of the central nervous system secondary to chimeric antigen receptor (CAR) T-cell therapy and conventional chemotherapy.

OVERVIEW

Medical therapies and interventions to improve patient morbidity and mortality can result in inadvertent neurologic sequelae. Recently, there has been much attention given to adverse effects secondary to antineoplastic therapies, as demonstrated by newly released National Institute of Health Cancer Moonshot Initiatives, one of which is to "minimize debilitating side effects of cancer and its treatment."[1] This review focuses on the histologic features and underlying mechanisms of the neuropathology associated with 2 types of

---

Department of Pathology, Brigham and Women's Hospital, Harvard Medical School, 75 Francis Street, Boston, MA 02115, USA
* Corresponding author.
E-mail address: mel_feany@hms.harvard.edu

Surgical Pathology 13 (2020) 331–342
https://doi.org/10.1016/j.path.2020.01.004

antineoplastic therapies—chimeric antigen receptor (CAR) T-cell therapy and conventional chemotherapy.

CAR T-CELL THERAPY

> ### Highlights
>
> Clinical:
>
> - Anti-CD19 chimeric antigen receptor (CAR) T-cell therapies show impressive, sustained therapeutic responses to several hematologic malignancies and are Food and Drug Administration approved for relapsed/refractory B-cell acute lymphoblastic leukemia and diffuse large B-cell lymphoma.
>
> - Adverse effects include cytokine release syndrome (CRS) and neurotoxicity (immune effector cell–associated neurotoxicity syndrome [ICANS]).
>
> Putative Mechanism of ICANS:
>
> - Expansion of CAR T cells after infusion results in release of cytokines, particularly from monocytes/macrophages. Elevated circulating cytokines likely cause endothelial activation and breakdown of the blood-brain barrier (BBB). Additional cytokines may be released from intracranial cell populations (eg, microglia, astrocytes, pericytes, and endothelial cells), potentially exacerbating BBB dysfunction.
>
> Histology:
>
> - Expansion of the perivascular spaces from extravasated fluid, vacuolated/degenerated white matter, gliosis, clasmatodendrosis, platelet microthrombi, fibrinoid vascular necrosis, hemorrhage, microinfarcts, and prominent/activated microglia have been observed in the more acute to subacute setting of ICANS.
>
> - Chronic changes may include gliosis, activated microglia, corpora amylacea, expansion of the perivascular space, evidence of remote hemorrhage, and cortical atrophy.
>
> - Inflammatory cell infiltrates (including CAR T cells, non-CAR T cells, and macrophages) are variable in extent and distribution (eg, perivascular, subarachnoid, meningeal, or intraparenchymal).
>
> - CRS in the absence of ICANS does not seem to have any overt, specific microscopic neuropathology.
>
> Histologic Differential:
>
> - Posterior reversible encephalopathy syndrome, viral encephalitis, cerebral malaria, acute necrotizing encephalopathy, acute hemorrhagic encephalopathy, and environmental toxins, among others.

Chimeric antigen receptor (CAR) T cells are a form of cancer immunotherapy in which autologous or allogenic T lymphocytes are engineered to express recombinant receptors composed of a tumor recognition region, a T-cell receptor intracellular signaling domain, and typically at least one intervening costimulatory domain. Recognition of the target antigen results in activation and proliferation of CAR T cells, leading to release of cytokines and tumor cell apoptosis. Although CAR T cells have been constructed to recognize several different tumor antigens, including mesothelin, Her2, B-cell maturation antigen, and glypican 3, the most promising target has been CD19. Numerous studies have demonstrated that anti-CD19 CAR T cells can produce significant and sustained therapeutic responses in patients with relapsed/refractory B-cell acute lymphoblastic leukemia, B-cell non-Hodgkin lymphoma, and chronic lymphocytic leukemia.[2–8] Reflecting the clinical efficacy of CAR T-cell therapy, the Food and Drug Administration has approved 2 anti-CD19 CAR T-cell products: tisagenlecleucel for use in refractory/relapsed B-ALL or diffuse large B-cell lymphoma (DLBCL) and axicabtagene ciloleucel for use in refractory/relapsed DLBCL.[9]

Despite their therapeutic utility, CAR T cells are associated with several complications such as cytokine release syndrome (CRS) and neurotoxicity (immune effector cell–associated neurotoxicity syndrome [ICANS]). CRS, which can be seen in 35% to 93% of patients receiving CAR T cells, usually manifests as fever and flu-like symptoms, although severe CRS can present as multiorgan failure, capillary leak syndrome, and hemodynamic instability; patients may show laboratory evidence of disseminated intravascular coagulation or overlap with macrophage activation syndrome/hemophagocytic lymphohistiocytosis.[10]

ICANS can manifest as encephalopathy, headache, tremor, ataxia, facial nerve palsy, seizures, and, in rare cases, fatal fulminant cerebral edema.[11,12] Incidence, severity, and timing of ICANS may vary by CAR T-cell infusion dose, lymphodepletion regimen, and patient age, among other clinical factors.[13] Although most patients with ICANS have history of CRS,[12] ICANS and CRS can occur independently of each other,[11] suggesting that these might be related but distinct phenomenon.

The mechanism underlying ICANS is still being elucidated, but recent advances have implicated a central role of circulating cytokines, endothelial activation, and blood-brain barrier (BBB) dysfunction. Histologic examination of animal models and postmortem human brain tissue has provided invaluable insight into the pathophysiology of this disorder. The authors now discuss the putative mechanism of ICANS.

Elevated circulating cytokines have been linked to ICANS. As previously mentioned, most of the patients with severe ICANS will have history of CRS,[3,7,8,12–14] and increased levels of circulating cytokines such as interkeukin (IL) 6, IL-2, IL-10, IL-15, interferon (IFN) γ, tumor necrosis factor alpha (TNFα), and granulocyte-macrophage colony-stimulating factor (CSF) have been correlated with the presence or severity of ICANS.[5,7,8,13,14] Elevated serum cytokines have also been shown in an anti-CD20 CAR T-cell nonhuman primate model demonstrating neurotoxicity.[15] Recent evidence from CAR T-cell mouse models[16,17] suggests that monocytes/macrophages (rather than CAR T cells) are the primary source of proinflammatory cytokines that account for the severity of CRS and ICANS. Macrophage depletion can abrogate CRS-related toxicity and release of IL-6.[18]

Elevated circulating cytokines may promote ICANS through aberrant endothelial activation and BBB dysfunction. Exposure to proinflammatory cytokines shifts endothelial cells from a quiescent to activated phenotype, a process that is mediated by the angiopoietin (ANG)–TIE2 system.[19,20] On activation, endothelial cells release ANG2 and von Willebrand factor (vWF) from storage granules called Weibel-Palade bodies into circulation.[19,21] ANG2 antagonizes ANG1-TIE2 signaling, disrupting endothelial quiescence and maturation, promoting leukocyte transmigration, and increasing BBB permeability via internalization of proteins necessarily for BBB integrity, such as tight junctions and adherens junctions.[19,22] Patients with severe ICANS show increased serum ANG2, reduced serum ANG1, and/or higher ANG2:ANG1 ratios,[8,13] providing biomarker evidence for endothelial activation. Moreover, patients with severe ICANS have elevated serum vWF and evidence of consumptive coagulopathy,[8,13] also in keeping with endothelial activation. Increased BBB permeability is supported by elevated CSF protein, CSF/serum albumin quotient, and proinflammatory cytokines in the CSF of patients with ICANS.[8,13] Elevated proinflammatory cytokines in the CSF have also

been demonstrated in a nonhuman primate model.[15]

Postmortem neuropathologic studies performed on CAR T-cell patients and animal models provide corroborating evidence for endothelial activation and BBB dysfunction. Gust and colleagues[13] reported platelet microthrombi, intravascular vWF binding, endothelial disruption, erythrocyte extravasation, microhemorrhages, and microinfarcts accompanied by vascular fibrinoid necrosis in a patient with severe ICANS who died 13 days after CAR T-cell infusion; platelet microthrombi were also identified in a second patient with history of severe ICANS. A case report of a patient who died from fulminant cerebral edema 4 days after CAR T-cell infusion (**Fig. 1**A, B) described expansion of the perivascular spaces (**Fig. 1**C) with fibrin and factor VIIIA-positive fluid (**Fig. 1**D), edematous, vacuolated white matter, and clasmatodendrosis (ie, beading and fragmentation of astrocytic processes), which was accentuated around blood vessels, consistent with BBB disruption (**Fig. 1**E).[23] A nonhuman primate model showed rare foci of perivascular edema during peak neurotoxicity.[15]

In addition, most histologic descriptions of ICANS comment on an inflammatory cell infiltrate involving central nervous system (CNS) tissue, compatible with altered BBB integrity. Descriptions from human and animal models include perivascular CD8+ lymphocytes, with the majority composed of CAR T cells[13]; intraparenchymal CD8+ T cells and abundant macrophages in degenerated white matter[6]; multifocal meningitis and perivascular and intraparenchymal T cells (both CAR T cells and non-CAR T cells)[15]; thickening of the meninges with infiltration of the subarachnoid space by macrophages[17]; and perivascular macrophages with only rare scattered lymphocytes (**Fig. 1**F, G) and no identifiable CAR T cells.[23] The variability in the number, composition, and distribution of inflammatory cells in the CNS raises questions about their role in the development of ICANS, particularly the role of infiltrating CAR T cells.

Cytokines may be relatively enriched in the CSF compared with peripheral blood during severe ICANS,[8,15,24] suggesting that there might be intracranial sources of cytokine production. Microglia are a possible candidate for intracranial production of cytokines,[25] and postmortem studies of patients with history of ICANS have consistently shown prominent and/or reactive microglia[6,13,23] (**Fig. 1**H). However, activated microglia or increased numbers of microglia have not been described in CAR T-cell animal models

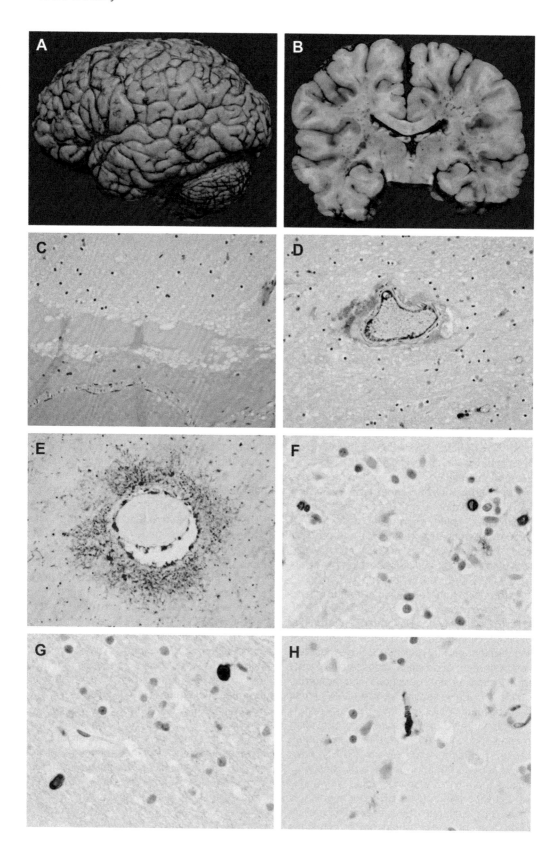

demonstrating neurotoxicity,[15,17] with one mouse model actually showing a reduction in the total number of Tmem119+ microglia compared with controls.[26] Other possible intracranial sources of cytokine production include pericytes,[13,27] endothelial cells,[22,28] and astrocytes.[29,30] Notably, release of cytokines by intracranial cell populations may further increase BBB permeability and exposure to circulating proinflammatory cytokines, resulting in a positive feedback loop that exacerbates BBB dysregulation.

Alterations of the cellular milieu of the CNS due to increased BBB permeability and exposure to elevated cytokines may be injurious to astrocytes and neurons. Elevation of CSF levels of S100 calcium-binding protein B and glial fibrillary acidic protein (GFAP) in patients with ICANS[14] and perivascular clasmatodendrosis in a postmortem examination of a patient with fatal CAR T-cell cerebral edema[23] suggest astrocyte injury. Diffuse gliosis, reflective of general CNS injury, has been reported.[6] Increased CSF concentrations of N-methyl-D-aspartate receptor agonists quinolinic acid and glutamate, compatible with excitotoxicity, have also been shown in patients with ICANS.[8] Exposure to excitotoxic agents may result in neuronal death.[31] Neuronal loss has been identified in the postmortem examination of one patient with history of optic atrophy and follicular lymphoma treated with CAR T-cell therapy and fludarabine lymphodepletion,[6] although the pathogenesis underlying this patient's neuronal loss is unclear and likely multifactorial.

Chronic changes associated with CAR T-cell therapy may include cortical atrophy, gliosis of the gray and white matter (particularly prominent in the subpial region), persistent microglial activation, widened perivascular spaces with hemosiderin-laden macrophages, and abundant corpora amylacea.[14]

Importantly, there does not seem to be overt, specific neuropathology associated with CRS in the absence of ICANS in individuals given CAR T-cell therapy. However, this observation is based on rare published descriptions. The gross and microscopic neuropathologic examination of one patient with severe CRS, but no history of ICANS, was described as grossly (**Fig. 2**A, B) and microscopically (**Fig. 2**C, D) unremarkable.[12] In a CAR T-cell mouse model showing CRS without neurotoxicity, there was no cerebral edema, gliosis, hemorrhage, or necrosis.[16]

To summarize, although the precise mechanism underlying ICANS is still being elucidated, there is an emerging model in which activation and expansion of CAR T cells result in cytokine release, particularly from monocytes/macrophages, inducing endothelial cell activation and BBB dysfunction. Cytokines can then cross the permeable BBB, which may also potentiate release of additional cytokines from pericytes, endothelial cells, astrocytes, and/or microglia in a positive feedback loop, further exacerbating BBB dysfunction. Exposure to cytokines may initiate cascades of events that are injurious to astrocytes and neurons. Neuropathologic examination of patients and animal models has shown a broad spectrum of histologic changes in association with ICANS, including perivascular fluid extravasation, platelet microthrombi, hemorrhage, microinfarcts, clasmatodendrosis, gliosis, microglial activation, and infiltration of the brain parenchyma, subarachnoid space, meninges, and/or perivascular spaces by inflammatory cells, including CAR T cells.

A diverse set of disorders may have histologic features that overlap with ICANS: posterior reversible encephalopathy syndrome (PRES) (which can be secondary to autoimmune disorders, hypertension, sepsis, amphetamine, and myriad medications including vascular endothelial growth factor inhibitors), viral encephalitis, cerebral malaria, acute necrotizing encephalopathy, acute hemorrhagic encephalopathy, and toxin exposure (eg, lead), among other entities. Correlation with clinical history and laboratory findings is essential for this histologic differential, especially because the microscopic features of ICANS are nonspecific and based on a limited number of published reports.

Fig. 1. Gross and microscopic neuropathologic findings in an anti-CD19 CAR T-cell patient with fulminant cerebral edema and severe ICANS. (*A*) Grossly edematous brain with (*B*) narrowed ventricles. There was (*C*) expansion of the perivascular spaces (H&E, 400x) with fibrin (not shown) and (*D*) factor-VIIIA-positive material (400x), consistent with fluid extravasation. (*E*) Clasmatodendrosis was particularly notable around blood vessels (GFAP, 400x), which suggests astrocyte injury and BBB dysfunction. (*F*) Admixed inflammatory cells were present (leukocyte common antigen stain, 1000x), including (*G*) scattered T cells (CD3, 1000x) and (*H*) activated rod microglia (CD68, 1000x). ICANS, immune effector cell–associated neurotoxicity syndrome.

CONVENTIONAL CHEMOTHERAPY

Highlights

Clinical:

- Neurologic adverse effects of conventional chemotherapy include encephalopathy, headache, neurovascular complications, seizures, movement disorders, pancerebellar syndrome, "stroke-like" syndrome, posterior reversible encephalopathy syndrome, chemotherapy-related cognitive impairment (CRCI), peripheral neuropathy, myopathy, and dysfunction of the enteric nervous system.

- Chemotherapy-induced leukoencephalopathy is particularly associated with methotrexate (although it has been observed with other chemotherapeutics), concurrent brain radiation, and intrathecal or intraventricular administration of chemotherapy.

- CRCI affects approximately 15% to 25% of patients, involves multiple cognitive domains, and may persist for up to 20 years after cessation of treatment in a subset of patients.

Putative Mechanism of Neurotoxicity Associated with Chemotherapy:

- Chemotherapy-induced leukoencephalopathy: the pathophysiology is unclear, but chemotherapeutic agents have a direct cytotoxic effect on central nervous system (CNS) progenitor cells and oligodendrocytes and impair the self-renewal potential of oligodendrocyte precursors at sublethal concentrations. Oxidative stress may also be contributory.

- CRCI: multiple implicated mechanisms include elevated proinflammatory cytokines, reactive oxygen species/oxidative stress, DNA damage, blood-brain barrier dysfunction, direct effects of chemotherapy on CNS cells, neuroinflammation, and dysmyelination.

Histology:

- Chemotherapy-induced leukoencephalopathy: foci of demyelination and necrosis, axonal swellings, myelin pallor, white matter vacuolization/spongiosis, edema, and gliosis, with a generally limited inflammatory cell reaction.

- CRCI: reactive astrocytes, activated microglia, reduced CNS progenitors, and oligodendrocytes.

Histologic Differential:

- Chemotherapy-induced leukoencephalopathy: leukoencephalopathy from another

inciting cause (eg, hypoxia, radiation, other therapeutic medication, metabolic disorder, AIDS, drugs of abuse, or environmental toxins), genetic leukodystrophy, demyelinating disorders, and infection (eg, JC virus).

Chemotherapeutic agents can be divided into several major classes based on mechanism of action and derivation, including alkylating agents, anthracyclines, antimetabolites, plant alkaloids, and topoisomerase inhibitors. Chemotherapy is associated with a range of adverse effects involving the CNS (eg, encephalopathy, headache, neurovascular complications, seizures, movement disorders, pancerebellar syndrome, "stroke-like" syndrome, PRES, and chemotherapy-related cognitive impairment [CRCI]), peripheral nervous system (eg, peripheral neuropathy), musculoskeletal system (eg, myopathy), and enteric nervous system. These adverse neurologic effects are clinically significant, can be dose-limiting, and may prompt cessation of therapy.

White matter damage following chemotherapy treatment (with or without radiation therapy) may manifest in severity from progressive and oftentimes fatal disseminated necrotizing leukoencephalopathy (DNL)[32] to transient, clinically asymptomatic lesions.[33] Although chemotherapy-induced leukoencephalopathy is commonly associated with methotrexate,[32,34,35] it has also been observed with fludarabine, carmustine, vincristine, cyclophosphamide, doxorubicin, 5-fluorouracil, and cisplatin, among other chemotherapeutic agents.[32,35–37] Intrathecal or intraventricular administration of chemotherapeutic agents and/or concurrent brain radiation may predispose patients to developing leukoencephalopathy.[32,34,35]

There is variability in the histologic descriptions of chemotherapy-induced leukoencephalopathy.[32,34–37] The prominent features of DNL[32] are multiple foci of demyelination and necrosis, often confluent and sometimes markedly extensive, with characteristic axonal swellings (composed of mitochondria, microfilaments, autophagic vacuoles, and calcifications) that are found within and adjacent to the foci of necrosis. Spongiosis, edema, and reactive astrocytes may be observed near the areas of demyelination and necrosis. Fibrinoid vascular necrosis and fibrin extravasation can be present but are most likely attributable to concurrent brain radiation. The accompanying inflammatory cell reaction is generally very limited. However, there may be abundant periodic acid–Schiff-positive macrophages.[36] The extent of myelin loss, white matter vacuolization, edema, gliosis, and

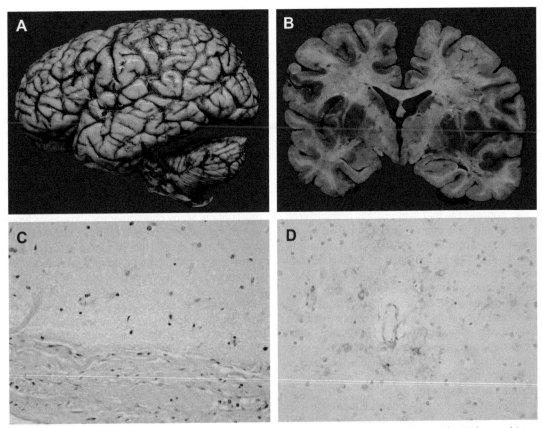

Fig. 2. Gross and microscopic neuropathologic findings in an anti-CD19 CAR T-cell patient with CRS but no history of ICANS. (*A, B*) Grossly unremarkable brain with (*C*) no specific microscopic pathologic change (H&E, 400x) and (*D*) minimal gliosis (GFAP, 400x).CRS, cytokine release syndrome; ICANS, immune effector cell–associated neurotoxicity syndrome.

frequency of axonal swellings in chemotherapy-induced leukoencephalopathy is highly variable.[36–38] An example of the histologic changes seen with a case of chemotherapy-induced leukoencephalopathy is provided in **Fig. 3**.

The histologic differential for chemotherapy-induced leukoencephalopathy is broad and includes leukoencephalopathy due to hypoxia, radiation, other therapeutic medication, metabolic disorder, AIDS, JC virus, drugs of abuse, or

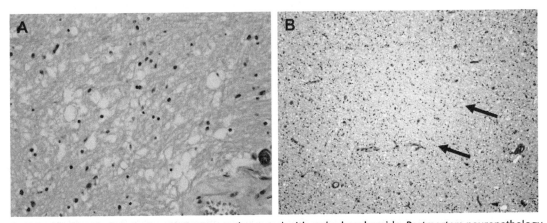

Fig. 3. Leukoencephalopathy in a patient recently treated with cyclophosphamide. Postmortem neuropathology was notable for (*A*) vacuolization of the white matter (H&E, 400x) with (*B*) subtle patchy loss of myelin (*arrows*, LFB/PAS, 100X).

environmental toxins; genetic leukodystrophy; and demyelinating disorders. Clinical history and laboratory findings will narrow the differential, as the histology can be nonspecific.

The pathophysiology of chemotherapy-induced leukoencephalopathy is unclear, but direct cytotoxicity of chemotherapy to CNS progenitor cells and oligodendrocytes is plausible. Neuronal and oligodendrocyte precursors, as well as oligodendrocytes, are extremely sensitive to multiple chemotherapeutic agents, even at low subtherapeutic concentrations.[39,40] Carmustine, lomustine, temozolomide, cisplatin, paclitaxel, and 5-fluorouracil have all been shown to cross the BBB.[41–44] It is also conceivable that systemically administered chemotherapeutic agents with poor BBB penetrance may accumulate at sufficient concentrations in the CNS to be lethal to CNS precursor cells and oligodendrocytes, particularly when there is compromise of BBB integrity as can be observed following brain radiation. In addition to their direct cytotoxic effects, chemotherapies may induce differentiation and persistent alterations in the self-renewal potential of oligodendrocyte precursors, potentially resulting in delayed myelination damage and impaired ability to repair subsequent white matter injury.[39,40,45] The presence of axonal swellings suggests impaired axonal transport, which may be mediated by direct action of certain chemotherapies on microtubules[46] or by oxidative stress/mitochondrial dysfunction.[47]

An increasingly recognized adverse neurologic effect of chemotherapy is the development of cognitive deficits (CRCI, sometimes referred to as "chemobrain" or "chemofog"). CRCI is observed in a subset of chemotherapy patients, typically cited in the range of 15% to 25%,[48] although the incidence may approach 80%.[49] Cognitive domains frequently impaired include memory, attention, executive function, and processing speed.[50] Although the extent of cognitive impairment may be mild to moderate[51] and vary depending on study design, patient characteristics, control group, cognitive domains examined, and whether baseline cognition is assessed,[52,53] these deficits are nevertheless associated with significant patient morbidity. Patients' perceived cognitive impairment may contribute to worse qualitative work-related outcomes[54] and impaired quality of life and daily functioning.[55] The incidence and severity of CRCI is generally thought to abate over time, but some patients have cognitive deficits that persist for up to 20 years after the last dose of chemotherapy,[56] and other patients only develop cognitive problems over a year after treatment cessation.[57] Radiologic studies have shown volumetric brain loss,[58,59] altered levels of brain activation during cognitive tasks,[60,61] evidence of impaired global brain network organization,[62] and changes to white matter integrity[63,64] following chemotherapy treatment. Older age, lower cognitive reserve, ApoE status, and other clinical factors may predispose patients to developing CRCI.[65,66]

The pathophysiology underlying CRCI is not fully elucidated, but data support several complementary mechanisms, including (1) elevated proinflammatory cytokines, reactive oxygen species (ROS), oxidative stress, and DNA damage; (2) BBB dysfunction; (3) direct effects of chemotherapy on CNS cells; (4) neuroinflammation; (5) and dysmyelination. Many chemotherapeutic agents function therapeutically by promoting oxidative stress and DNA damage.[67] This is done through several pathways such as generation of superoxide radicals and ROS.[68] Patients treated with chemotherapy have increased circulating ROS.[69] Chemotherapy is also associated with elevated peripheral proinflammatory cytokines,[70–73] such as IL-6 and TNFα, that are released from inflammatory cells,[74] tumor cells,[75] and nonneoplastic tissue including gastrointestinal mucosa.[76] Peripheral ROS and proinflammatory cytokines can alter the permeability of the BBB,[77] potentially allowing greater concentrations of chemotherapeutic agents and peripheral cytokines to cross the BBB into the brain, which has several important sequelae. Firstly, the direct effects of chemotherapy on CNS progenitor cells and oligodendrocytes[39,40] may contribute not only to white matter damage but also to impaired hippocampal neurogenesis and memory deficits.[39,78–80] Secondly, circulating proinflammatory cytokines and ROS can instigate neuroinflammation, leading to increased intracranial production of cytokines, mitochondrial dysfunction,[81] oxidative stress,[82] and neuron apoptosis.[83] Neuroinflammation also impairs hippocampal neurogenesis.[84] Data from Gibson and colleagues[85] support a central role of microglia in the cognitive deficits, induction of astrocyte reactivity, altered oligodendrocyte lineage dynamics, and reduced myelin sheath thickness in their mouse model of CRCI.

SUMMARY

Iatrogenic neuropathology secondary to systemic antineoplastic agents such as CAR T-cell therapy and conventional chemotherapy may result in significant patient morbidity and mortality. Understanding the pathophysiology underlying these adverse effects not only offers insight into potential ameliorating therapies but also sheds light on the regulation of the neurovascular unit and how circulating cytokines and other substances may either impair or directly cross the BBB, initiating cascades of deleterious, sometimes chronic, effects potentially mediated by cell populations intrinsic to the CNS. These pathways may be relevant to neurodegeneration and senescence of the aging brain.

DISCLOSURE

The authors have no sources of funding to disclose. The authors declare no conflict of interest.

REFERENCES

1. Cancer Moonshot[SM] Research Initiatives. Available at: https://www.cancer.gov/research/key-initiatives/moonshot-cancer-initiative/implementation. Accessed August 20, 2019.
2. Maude SL, Frey N, Shaw PA, et al. Chimeric antigen receptor T cells for sustained remissions in leukemia. N Engl J Med 2014;371(16):1507–17.
3. Maude SL, Laetsch TW, Buechner J, et al. Tisagenlecleucel in Children and Young Adults with B-Cell Lymphoblastic Leukemia. N Engl J Med 2018;378(5):439–48.
4. Locke FL, Neelapu SS, Bartlett NL, et al. Phase 1 Results of ZUMA-1: A Multicenter Study of KTE-C19 Anti-CD19 CAR T Cell Therapy in Refractory Aggressive Lymphoma. MolTher 2017;25(1):285–95.
5. Neelapu SS, Locke FL, Bartlett NL, et al. AxicabtageneCiloleucel CAR T-Cell Therapy in Refractory Large B-Cell Lymphoma. N Engl J Med 2017;377(26):2531–44.
6. Schuster SJ, Svoboda J, Chong EA, et al. Chimeric Antigen Receptor T Cells in Refractory B-Cell Lymphomas. N Engl J Med 2017;377(26):2545–54.
7. Turtle CJ, Hay KA, Hanafi LA, et al. Durable Molecular Remissions in Chronic Lymphocytic Leukemia Treated With CD19-Specific Chimeric Antigen Receptor-Modified T Cells After Failure of Ibrutinib. J ClinOncol 2017;35(26):3010–20.
8. Santomasso BD, Park JH, Salloum D, et al. Clinical and Biological Correlates of Neurotoxicity Associated with CAR T-cell Therapy in Patients with B-cell Acute Lymphoblastic Leukemia. CancerDiscov 2018;8(8):958–71.
9. Boyiadzis MM, Dhodapkar MV, Brentjens RJ, et al. Chimeric antigen receptor (CAR) T therapies for the treatment of hematologic malignancies: clinical perspective and significance. J ImmunotherCancer 2018;6(1):137.
10. Hirayama AV, Turtle CJ. Toxicities of CD19 CAR-T cell immunotherapy. Am J Hematol 2019;94(S1):S42–9.
11. Brudno JN, Kochenderfer JN. Toxicities of chimeric antigen receptor T cells: recognition and management. Blood 2016;127(26):3321–30.
12. Rubin DB, Danish HH, Ali AB, et al. Neurological toxicities associated with chimeric antigen receptor T-cell therapy. Brain 2019;142(5):1334–48.
13. Gust J, Hay KA, Hanafi LA, et al. Endothelial Activation and Blood-Brain Barrier Disruption in Neurotoxicity after Adoptive Immunotherapy with CD19 CAR-T Cells. CancerDiscov 2017;7(12):1404–19.
14. Gust J, Finney OC, Li D, et al. Glial injury in neurotoxicity after pediatric CD19-directed chimeric antigen receptor T cell therapy. Ann Neurol 2019;86(1):42–54.
15. Taraseviciute A, Tkachev V, Ponce R, et al. Chimeric Antigen Receptor T Cell-Mediated Neurotoxicity in Nonhuman Primates. CancerDiscov 2018;8(6):750–63.
16. Giavridis T, van der Stegen SJC, Eyquem J, et al. CAR T cell-induced cytokine release syndrome is mediated by macrophages and abated by IL-1 blockade. Nat Med 2018;24(6):731–8.
17. Norelli M, Camisa B, Barbiera G, et al. Monocyte-derived IL-1 and IL-6 are differentially required for cytokine-release syndrome and neurotoxicity due to CAR T cells. Nat Med 2018;24(6):739–48.
18. van der Stegen SJ, Davies DM, Wilkie S, et al. Preclinical in vivo modeling of cytokine release syndrome induced by ErbB-retargeted human T cells: identifying a window of therapeutic opportunity? J Immunol 2013;191(9):4589–98.
19. Augustin HG, Koh GY, Thurston G, et al. Control of vascular morphogenesis and homeostasis through the angiopoietin-Tie system. Nat Rev MolCell Biol 2009;10(3):165–77.
20. Fiedler U, Reiss Y, Scharpfenecker M, et al. Angiopoietin-2 sensitizes endothelial cells to TNF-alpha and has a crucial role in the induction of inflammation. Nat Med 2006;12(2):235–9.
21. Rondaij MG, Bierings R, Kragt A, et al. Dynamics and plasticity of Weibel-Palade bodies in endothelial cells. ArteriosclerThrombVasc Biol 2006;26(5):1002–7.
22. Blecharz-Lang KG, Wagner J, Fries A, et al. Interleukin 6-mediated endothelial barrier disturbances can be attenuated by blockade of the IL6 receptor expressed in brain microvascular endothelial cells. TranslStroke Res 2018;9(6):631–42.
23. Torre M, Solomon IH, Sutherland CL, et al. Neuropathology of a case with fatal CAR T-cell-associated cerebral edema. J NeuropatholExp Neurol 2018;77(10):877–82.
24. Hu Y, Sun J, Wu Z, et al. Predominant cerebral cytokine release syndrome in CD19-directed chimeric antigen receptor-modified T cell therapy. J HematolOncol 2016;9(1):70.

25. Hanisch UK. Microglia as a source and target of cytokines. Glia 2002;40(2):140–55.

26. Pennell CA, Barnum JL, McDonald-Hyman CS, et al. Human CD19-targeted mouse T cells induce B cell aplasia and toxicity in human CD19 transgenic mice. MolTher 2018;26(6):1423–34.

27. Guijarro-Muñoz I, Compte M, Álvarez-Cienfuegos A, et al. Lipopolysaccharide activates Toll-like receptor 4 (TLR4)-mediated NF-κB signaling pathway and proinflammatory response in human pericytes. J Biol Chem 2014;289(4):2457–68.

28. Vadeboncoeur N, Segura M, Al-Numani D, et al. Pro-inflammatory cytokine and chemokine release by human brain microvascular endothelial cells stimulated by Streptococcus suis serotype 2. FEMSImmunol Med Microbiol 2003;35(1):49–58.

29. Lieberman AP, Pitha PM, Shin HS, et al. Production of tumor necrosis factor and other cytokines by astrocytes stimulated with lipopolysaccharide or a neurotropic virus. ProcNatlAcadSciUS A 1989; 86(16):6348–52.

30. Sofroniew MV. Multiple roles for astrocytes as effectors of cytokines and inflammatory mediators. Neuroscientist 2014;20(2):160–72.

31. Sattler R, Tymianski M. Molecular mechanisms of glutamate receptor-mediated excitotoxic neuronal cell death. MolNeurobiol 2001;24(1–3):107–29.

32. Rubinstein LJ, Herman MM, Long TF, et al. Disseminated necrotizing leukoencephalopathy: a complication of treated central nervous system leukemia and lymphoma. Cancer 1975;35(2):291–305.

33. Fouladi M, Chintagumpala M, Laningham FH, et al. White matter lesions detected by magnetic resonance imaging after radiotherapy and high-dose chemotherapy in children with medulloblastoma or primitive neuroectodermal tumor. J ClinOncol 2004; 22(22):4551–60.

34. Lai R, Abrey LE, Rosenblum MK, et al. Treatment-induced leukoencephalopathy in primary CNS lymphoma: a clinical and autopsy study. Neurology 2004;62(3):451–6.

35. Robain O, Dulac O, Dommergues JP, et al. Necrotisingleukoencephalopathy complicating treatment of childhood leukaemia. J NeurolNeurosurgPsychiatry 1984;47(1):65–72.

36. Spriggs DR, Stopa E, Mayer RJ, et al. Fludarabine phosphate (NSC 312878) infusions for the treatment of acute leukemia: phase I and neuropathological study. Cancer Res 1986;46(11):5953–8.

37. Moore-Maxwell CA, Datto MB, Hulette CM. Chemotherapy-induced toxic leukoencephalopathy causes a wide range of symptoms: a series of four autopsies. Mod Pathol 2004;17(2):241–7.

38. Moore BE, Somers NP, Smith TW. Methotrexate-related nonnecrotizing multifocal axonopathy detected by beta-amyloid precursor protein immunohistochemistry. Arch Pathol Lab Med 2002;126(1):79–81.

39. Dietrich J, Han R, Yang Y, et al. CNS progenitor cells and oligodendrocytes are targets of chemotherapeutic agents in vitro and in vivo. J Biol 2006;5(7):22.

40. Han R, Yang YM, Dietrich J, et al. Systemic 5-fluorouracil treatment causes a syndrome of delayed myelin destruction in the central nervous system. J Biol 2008;7(4):12.

41. Sawyer AJ, Piepmeier JM, Saltzman WM. New methods for direct delivery of chemotherapy for treating brain tumors. Yale J Biol Med 2006; 79(3–4):141–52.

42. Ginos JZ, Cooper AJ, Dhawan V, et al. [13N]cisplatin PET to assess pharmacokinetics of intra-arterial versus intravenous chemotherapy for malignant brain tumors. J Nucl Med 1987;28(12):1844–52.

43. Gangloff A, Hsueh WA, Kesner AL, et al. Estimation of paclitaxel biodistribution and uptake in human-derived xenografts in vivo with (18)F-fluoropaclitaxel. J Nucl Med 2005;46(11):1866–71.

44. Bourke RS, West CR, Chheda G, et al. Kinetics of entry and distribution of 5-fluorouracil in cerebrospinal fluid and brain following intravenous injection in a primate. Cancer Res 1973;33(7):1735–46.

45. Hyrien O, Dietrich J, Noble M. Mathematical and experimental approaches to identify and predict the effects of chemotherapy on neuroglial precursors. Cancer Res 2010;70(24):10051–9.

46. Tanner KD, Levine JD, Topp KS. Microtubule disorientation and axonal swelling in unmyelinated sensory axons during vincristine-induced painful neuropathy in rat. J Comp Neurol 1998;395(4):481–92.

47. Fang C, Bourdette D, Banker G. Oxidative stress inhibits axonal transport: implications for neurodegenerative diseases. MolNeurodegener 2012;7:29.

48. Ahles TA, Root JC, Ryan EL. Cancer- and cancer treatment-associated cognitive change: an update on the state of the science. J ClinOncol 2012; 30(30):3675–86.

49. Wefel JS, Schagen SB. Chemotherapy-related cognitive dysfunction. CurrNeurolNeurosci Rep 2012;12(3):267–75.

50. Pendergrass JC, Targum SD, Harrison JE. Cognitive Impairment Associated with Cancer: A Brief Review. InnovClinNeurosci 2018;15(1–2):36–44.

51. Falleti MG, Sanfilippo A, Maruff P, et al. The nature and severity of cognitive impairment associated with adjuvant chemotherapy in women with breast cancer: a meta-analysis of the current literature. BrainCogn 2005;59(1):60–70.

52. Bernstein LJ, McCreath GA, Komeylian Z, et al. Cognitive impairment in breast cancer survivors treated with chemotherapy depends on control group type and cognitive domains assessed: A multilevel meta-analysis. NeurosciBiobehav Rev 2017;83:417–28.

53. Ono M, Ogilvie JM, Wilson JS, et al. A meta-analysis of cognitive impairment and decline associated with

adjuvant chemotherapy in women with breast cancer. Front Oncol 2015;5:59.

54. Bijker R, Duijts SFA, Smith SN, et al. Functional Impairments and Work-Related Outcomes in Breast Cancer Survivors: A Systematic Review. J OccupRehabil 2018;28(3):429–51.

55. Hutchinson AD, Hosking JR, Kichenadasse G, et al. Objective and subjective cognitive impairment following chemotherapy for cancer: a systematic review. Cancer Treat Rev 2012;38(7):926–34.

56. Koppelmans V, Breteler MM, Boogerd W, et al. Neuropsychological performance in survivors of breast cancer more than 20 years after adjuvant chemotherapy. J ClinOncol 2012;30(10):1080–6.

57. Wefel JS, Saleeba AK, Buzdar AU, et al. Acute and late onset cognitive dysfunction associated with chemotherapy in women with breast cancer. Cancer 2010;116(14):3348–56.

58. McDonald BC, Conroy SK, Ahles TA, et al. Gray matter reduction associated with systemic chemotherapy for breast cancer: a prospective MRI study. BreastCancer Res Treat 2010;123(3):819–28.

59. Koppelmans V, de Ruiter MB, van der Lijn F, et al. Global and focal brain volume in long-term breast cancer survivors exposed to adjuvant chemotherapy. BreastCancer Res Treat 2012;132(3):1099–106.

60. LópezZunini RA, Scherling C, Wallis N, et al. Differences in verbal memory retrieval in breast cancer chemotherapy patients compared to healthy controls: a prospective fMRI study. BrainImagingBehav 2013;7(4):460–77.

61. Conroy SK, McDonald BC, Smith DJ, et al. Alterations in brain structure and function in breast cancer survivors: effect of post-chemotherapy interval and relation to oxidative DNA damage. BreastCancer Res Treat 2013;137(2):493–502.

62. Bruno J, Hosseini SM, Kesler S. Altered resting state functional brain network topology in chemotherapy-treated breast cancer survivors. Neurobiol Dis 2012;48(3):329–38.

63. Deprez S, Amant F, Smeets A, et al. Longitudinal assessment of chemotherapy-induced structural changes in cerebral white matter and its correlation with impaired cognitive functioning. J ClinOncol 2012;30(3):274–81.

64. Deprez S, Amant F, Yigit R, et al. Chemotherapy-induced structural changes in cerebral white matter and its correlation with impaired cognitive functioning in breast cancer patients. Hum BrainMapp 2011;32(3):480–93.

65. Ahles TA, Saykin AJ, McDonald BC, et al. Longitudinal assessment of cognitive changes associated with adjuvant treatment for breast cancer: impact of age and cognitive reserve. J ClinOncol 2010;28(29):4434–40.

66. Mandelblatt JS, Small BJ, Luta G, et al. Cancer-related cognitive outcomes among older breast cancer survivors in the thinking and living with cancer study. J Clin Oncol 2018;36:3211–22.

67. Chen Y, Jungsuwadee P, Vore M, et al. Collateral damage in cancer chemotherapy: oxidative stress in nontargeted tissues. MolInterv 2007;7(3):147–56.

68. Conklin KA. Chemotherapy-associated oxidative stress: impact on chemotherapeutic effectiveness. IntegrCancerTher 2004;3(4):294–300.

69. Cetin T, Arpaci F, Yilmaz MI, et al. Oxidative stress in patients undergoing high-dose chemotherapy plus peripheral blood stem cell transplantation. BiolTrace Elem Res 2004;97(3):237–47.

70. Castel H, Denouel A, Lange M, et al. Biomarkers Associated with Cognitive Impairment in Treated Cancer Patients: Potential Predisposition and Risk Factors. Front Pharmacol 2017;8:138.

71. Kesler S, Janelsins M, Koovakkattu D, et al. Reduced hippocampal volume and verbal memory performance associated with interleukin-6 and tumor necrosis factor-alpha levels in chemotherapy-treated breast cancer survivors. BrainBehav Immun 2013;30(Suppl):S109–16.

72. Cheung YT, Ng T, Shwe M, et al. Association of proinflammatory cytokines and chemotherapy-associated cognitive impairment in breast cancer patients: a multi-centered, prospective, cohort study. Ann Oncol 2015;26(7):1446–51.

73. Pusztai L, Mendoza TR, Reuben JM, et al. Changes in plasma levels of inflammatory cytokines in response to paclitaxel chemotherapy. Cytokine 2004;25(3):94–102.

74. Aluise CD, Miriyala S, Noel T, et al. 2-Mercaptoethanesulfonate prevents doxorubicin-induced plasma protein oxidation and TNF-α release: implications for the reactive oxygen species-mediated mechanisms of chemobrain. FreeRadicBiol Med 2011;50(11):1630–8.

75. Edwardson DW, Boudreau J, Mapletoft J, et al. Inflammatory cytokine production in tumor cells upon chemotherapy drug exposure or upon selection for drug resistance. PLoS One 2017;12(9):e0183662.

76. Sonis ST. The pathobiology of mucositis. Nat Rev Cancer 2004;4(4):277–84.

77. Schreibelt G, Kooij G, Reijerkerk A, et al. Reactive oxygen species alter brain endothelial tight junction dynamics via RhoA, PI3 kinase, and PKB signaling. FASEB J 2007;21(13):3666–76.

78. Janelsins MC, Roscoe JA, Berg MJ, et al. IGF-1 partially restores chemotherapy-induced reductions in neural cell proliferation in adult C57BL/6 mice. Cancer Invest 2010;28(5):544–53.

79. Winocur G, Berman H, Nguyen M, et al. Neurobiological Mechanisms of Chemotherapy-induced Cognitive Impairment in a Transgenic Model of Breast Cancer. Neuroscience 2018;369:51–65.

80. Briones TL, Woods J. Chemotherapy-induced cognitive impairment is associated with decreases

in cell proliferation and histone modifications. BMCNeurosci 2011;12:124.

81. Tangpong J, Cole MP, Sultana R, et al. Adriamycin-induced, TNF-alpha-mediated central nervous system toxicity. Neurobiol Dis 2006;23(1):127–39.

82. Joshi G, Sultana R, Tangpong J, et al. Free radical mediated oxidative stress and toxic side effects in brain induced by the anti cancer drug adriamycin: insight into chemobrain. FreeRadic Res 2005; 39(11):1147–54.

83. Yuste JE, Tarragon E, Campuzano CM, et al. Implications of glial nitric oxide in neurodegenerative diseases. Front CellNeurosci 2015;9:322.

84. Chesnokova V, Pechnick RN, Wawrowsky K. Chronic peripheral inflammation, hippocampal neurogenesis, and behavior. BrainBehav Immun 2016;58:1–8.

85. Gibson EM, Nagaraja S, Ocampo A, et al. Methotrexate chemotherapy induces persistent tri-glial dysregulation that underlies chemotherapy-related cognitive impairment. Cell 2019;176(1–2):43–55.e13.

From Banding to BAM Files
Genomics Informs Diagnosis and Precision Medicine for Brain Tumors

Adrian M. Dubuc, PhD

KEYWORDS

- Central nervous system (CNS) • Brain tumors • Genomics • Epigenomics
- Next-generation sequencing • Cytogenetics

Key points

- Diagnosis of tumors of the central nervous system often necessitates evaluation of genomic features.
- Pediatric and adult brain tumors are characterized by distinct patterns of single nucleotide variants, copy-number alterations, epigenomic alterations, and/or structural rearrangements.
- No single genomic/epigenomic assay is currently suitable for all brain tumors; however, combinatorial use of cytogenetic and molecular methods can improve diagnosis and therapeutic management.

ABSTRACT

Tumors of the central nervous system (CNS) have been historically classified according to their morphologic and immunohistochemical features. In 2016, updates to the classification of tumors of the CNS by the World Health Organization revolutionized this paradigm. For the first time, genomic findings, whether whole-arm chromosomal aberrations or single nucleotide variants, represent a necessary and critical component of diagnosis, contributing or superseding histologic findings. These updates stem from decades of technical innovation and genomic discovery. During this time, there has been a dramatic expansion and evolution in clinical genomic assays for these tumors, informing diagnosis and guiding therapeutic management.

OVERVIEW

Tumors of the central nervous system (CNS) are highly heterogeneous in nature, demonstrating a diverse disease course from clinically benign to highly aggressive.[1] Patient stratification and disease management are predicated on accurate diagnosis. Although morphologic and immunohistochemical evaluation has long been espoused as a means of tumor classification, advances from the "omics" era have shed light on the inherent limitations of this approach.[2] Today, it is appreciated that tumors with similar morphologic appearance may demonstrate unique molecular features, highlighting their distinct genomic or epigenomic cause. In 2016, the World Health Organization (WHO) updated the classification of many CNS entities, for the first time incorporating genotypic features to the phenotypic diagnostic criteria.[3] These changes were implemented to more accurately define disease entities, in turn leading to improved patient management. Notably, these molecular markers include pathognomonic single nucleotide variants (SNVs), copy-number alterations, and structural rearrangements. Because there currently does not exist a single assay that can simultaneously and robustly interrogate this panoply of clinically significant genomic alterations,

---

The author has no sources of funding to disclose. The author declares no conflict of interest.
Department of Pathology, Harvard Medical School, Brigham and Women's Hospital, 75 Francis Street, Boston, MA 02115, USA
E-mail address: adubuc@bwh.harvard.edu

surgpath.theclinics.com

clinicians are required to understand the inherent strengths and weaknesses of the current modalities of testing to inform their ordering practices.

Clinical laboratory genetics has traditionally been divided into 2 broad categories: (1) cytogenetics, focused on the numerical and structural evaluation of chromosomes[4]; and (2) molecular genetics, evaluating the nature and structure of genes.[5] This divide was predicated on the divergence of both techniques and expertise required to perform analyses. Cytogenetics necessitated cell culture and microscopy techniques,[6] whereas molecular genetics emphasized polymerase chain reaction–based approaches.[5] Technological advances in laboratory medicine, largely driven by advances in sequence-based approaches, have forcefully begun to blur the once distinct boundaries between these fields.[7] Although laboratory genomics continues to evolve toward a single discipline, current approaches for cancer diagnostics remain largely centered on evaluating either cytogenetic or molecular genetic alterations. In the present review, the importance and limitations of cytogenetic and molecular genetic assays are described, highlighting their current and future potential.

EVOLUTION IN CYTOGENOMICS

Study of chromosome form and structure is intrinsically tied to lessons learned from karyotyping. In this modality of testing, cells are cultured in vitro, arrested in metaphase, and subsequently, chromosome are banded, permitting visual appreciation of both copy number and structural variation at a single-cell level.[7] For brain tumors, the use of karyotyping (first in a research setting) identified recurrent pattern of copy-number alterations, most often losses, associated with specific disease entities.[4,8] Many disease-specific chromosomal profiles identified during this era, including polysomy of chromosome 7 with concomitant loss of 9p and chromosome 10 described in gliomas, still hold true today.[4] Moreover, cytogenetics afforded us with a mechanistic understanding of oncogene activation or tumor suppressor gene disruption.[9] By example, the identification of small acentric extrachromosomal fragments, namely double minutes, as well as homogenous staining regions, is now well understood to represent a means through which oncogene amplification occurs,[9] a phenomenon well established and highly prevalent in glioblastoma associated with *EGFR* amplification.[10] Similarly, cytogenetic approaches can easily resolve changes to ploidy, including whole-genome doubling now thought to represent an independent predictor of poor prognosis across brain tumor entities,[11] or haploidy, associated with giant-cell glioblastoma.[4] Karyotyping, however, is plagued by significant limitations. Resolution of chromosome studies by standard Giemsa trypsin G-banding can only detect alterations greater than ~7 to 10 Mb. Moreover, and perhaps more significantly, karyotyping requires actively diving cells. As improvements in surgical methodologies have resulted in appropriately smaller biopsies, fresh tissue is often limited, and even when obtained, a normal result does not exclude the possibility of a neoplastic proliferation because outgrowth of normal tissue is not uncommon.[12] Despite its limitations, karyotyping is still used as a diagnostic assay in several clinical laboratories; however, its utility is rapidly diminishing and is increasingly being replaced by microarray and sequence-based approaches.

To overcome some of the inherent limitations of karyotyping, newer cytogenetic techniques, namely, fluorescence in situ hybridization (FISH), emerged. FISH studies use fluorescently labeled DNA probes, typically 150 to 500 kb in length, that bind DNA, to assess the copy number or structure of a specific genomic locus, or limited number of loci.[13] FISH studies can be performed on interphase nuclei and thus do not require cells to be actively dividing and can be adapted for both fresh or formalin-fixed paraffin embedded (FFPE) material. FISH studies are ideally suited for clinical scenarios in which a differential diagnosis necessitated the detection or exclusion of a specific structural rearrangement, such as BRAF rearrangement associated with pilocytic astrocytomas. Results can be achieved in 3 to 7 days from paraffin material, or within the 1 to 2 days for fresh tissue. Notably, most paraffin FISH studies are performed on 5-μm sections. When performed in this manner, the morphology and tissue architecture are retained. Areas of specific interest can thus be specifically evaluated.[13,14] Much like karyotyping, FISH provides single-cell analysis, thereby capturing intratumoral heterogeneity, evident in glioblastomas with EGFRvIII variant.[15] However, the targeted nature of FISH studies can lead to disconcerting and well-documented false positives. Most notably, confirmation of 1p/19q whole-arm co-deletion typically involved FISH-based assessment. The most common commercially available probe set used clinically evaluates the ratio of 1p to 1q versus the ratio of 19p to 19q to assess whole-arm co-deletion.[14] This indirect measure is problematic as IDH-mutant astrocytomas can, rarely, display subtelomeric deletions leading to false-positive 1p/19q deletion results using FISH studies.[16] As a result of this diagnostic pitfall, the WHO in fact recommends assays that can confirm the presence of whole-arm deletion for the diagnostic confirmation of oligodendroglioma.[3]

As a means of evaluating the genome-wide copy-number landscape, chromosomal microarray (CMA) is ideally suited. This assay involves DNA extraction and subsequent fragmentation. DNA molecules are labeled and hybridized onto a solid matrix.[7] The amount of labeled DNA that hybridizes to a specific probe (ie, feature) of the microarray generates a proportional signal, which can be normalized to a reference and subsequently converted into copy-number state.[7] The ability to accurately assess genome-wide copy-number aberrations can provide important and necessary support for diagnosis of gliomas, clearly delineating copy-number profiles associated with oligodendrogliomas versus those detected in astrocytomas and primary glioblastomas.[17,18] Similarly, for pediatric tumors such as medulloblastoma, a copy-number profile can support molecular subclassification, with admittedly variable success ranging from 47% to 79% of cases.[19] Technological improvements in both the probe density and the array design of CMAs have resulted in marked changes. With increased density, CMAs can now readily detect alterations often as small as ~50 kb, and optimized design facilitates use of DNA extracted from FFPE material.[20] CMA does not have the ability to identify evidence of balanced rearrangements[20]; however, intragenic copy-number alterations may be suggestive of unbalanced rearrangements. By example, the presence of 240-kb deletion on 6q22.1 partially encompassing the 5' region of ROS1 is now known to correlate an in-frame GOPC-ROS1 fusion, which may be responsive to targeted inhibition,[21,22] while a 1.9 Mb gain on 7q34 partially BRAF is known to be pathognomonic of KIAA1549-BRAF fusion.[19] CMA results are necessarily more complex than other cytogenetic testing, in part because of the increased resolution, which may impact the turn-around time in a clinical setting. Recently, guidelines have been described in an effort to achieve consistency in the manner in which CMAs results are reported.[23]

FROM SINGLE NUCLEOTIDE VARIANTS TO WHOLE-EXOME SEQUENCING

The rapid evolution of clinical laboratory genomics is perhaps no more evident than in the review of changes to sequencing approaches.

Sanger-based methods, in which DNA replications occur through use of dideoxynucleotides that cause chain termination, were traditionally used for the detection of gene-level alterations, most often in the form of SNVs.[24] Through capillary electrophoresis, fragments are sorted by length, and the underlying DNA sequence was obtained.[24] Sanger sequencing remains the gold standard in part because of the quality of data and the length of sequencing reads.[25] Rapidly, new approaches for sequencing were developed, including, but not limited to, pyrosequencing. Through pyrosequencing, genomic loci, often mutational hotspots, could be rapidly and cost-effectively evaluated.[14]

More recently, next-generation sequencing (NGS) approaches revolutionized the ease through which genomic information could be gathered. Gigabases of data could rapidly and cost-effectively be generated, which led to increased understanding of the underlying genomic complexity of many tumor types. Today, a vast array of both commercial and custom NGS approaches exists, which has been deployed clinically. These assays show tremendous versatility. They can be RNA or DNA based, amplicon derived versus capture based designed primarily for relatively rapid (3–7 day) analysis of SNVs and short insertion/deletions (indels) to whole-exome sequencing approaches. Although there is no single approach that has been universally adopted, many laboratories offer targeted panels with 150 to 500 genes that are known to be clinically important across many cancer types. Although this technology has tremendous capabilities, NGS has created a new bottleneck, often requiring extensive bioinformatics support, including generation of knowledge bases to facilitate rapid clinical interpretation. Beyond the single nucleotide alterations exists the potential to further extract mutational signature and copy-number aberrations from the data that are generated. Since the discovery of checkpoint inhibitor efficacy against multiple tumor types with mismatch repair deficiency,[26] assessment of increased tumor mutational burden and mutational signatures associated with inactivation of DNA repair machinery is becoming increasingly desired for treatment planning.[27] Furthermore, despite the limited genomic coverage of targeted platforms, the copy-number data extracted has the potential to be equivalent to that from CMA, potentially obviating dedicated copy-number analysis in most instances.[28]

EPIGENOMICS AS AN EMERGING DIAGNOSTIC TOOL

Recently, epigenetics, and specifically, DNA methylation patterns have been described as a robust means of confirming or supporting the histopathology diagnosis of CNS tumors.[29] DNA methylation patterns observed in these tumors are a reflection of its cellular origin, state of differentiation, and subsequent somatic alterations.[30] Methylation profiling is currently performed on both fresh and FFPE-derived specimens, in which extracted DNA is bisulfite converted and subsequently hybridized onto a microarray platform.[31] Bisulfite conversion deaminates unmethylated cytosines, resulting in conversion to uracil, whereas methylated residues are protected.[29] Profiling of large cohorts of tumors coupled with machine learning approaches was used to develop an epigenomic classifier, whose use was concordant with histopathology diagnosis in 88% of 1104 cases evaluated.[29] Notably, in the remaining 12% of cases, methylation-based studies resulted in revision of the histopathology diagnosis. Although this approach has the potential to clarify unusual cases, much of this work stems from a single-institutional experience and has not been widely adopted as a routine diagnostic tool in North America.

SUMMARY

Given the plurality of various testing modes that exist, and the absence of a uniform standard diagnostic approach, disease-specific testing algorithms have the potential to both confirm histopathology diagnosis when needed and identify possible actionable alterations for personalized medicine approaches. As molecular technologies and bioinformatics capabilities continue to improve, it is possible that a single, stand-alone assay will someday be able to deliver all clinically relevant genomic alterations for a given disease. For the time being, however, proper assay selection must necessarily be guided by clinical suspicion and treatment planning requirements.

REFERENCES

1. Archer TC, Sengupta S, Pomeroy SL. Brain cancer genomics and epigenomics. Handb Clin Neurol 2018. https://doi.org/10.1016/B978-0-444-64076-5.00050-8, 1st edition.
2. Van Den Bent MJ, Weller M, Wen PY, et al. A clinical perspective on the 2016 WHO brain tumor classification and routine molecular diagnostics. Neuro Oncol 2017;19:614–24.
3. Louis DN, Perry A, Reifenberger G, et al. The 2016 World Health Organization Classification of Tumors of the Central Nervous System: a summary. Acta Neuropathol 2016;131:803–20.
4. Bigner SH, Mark J, Friedman HS, et al. Structural chromosomal abnormalities in human medulloblastoma. Cancer Genet Cytogenet 1988;30:91–101. Available at: http://www.ncbi.nlm.nih.gov/pubmed/3422050.
5. Katsanis SH, Katsanis N. Molecular Genetic Testing and The Future of Clinical Genomics. Nat Rev Genet 2013;14(6):415–26. Available at: https://nam03.safelinks.protection.outlook.com/?url=https%3A%2F%2Fpubmed.ncbi.nlm.nih.gov%2F23681062%2F&data=02%7C01%7CJ.Surendrakumar%40elsevier.com%7C3d2286b260054f383aac08d7eacbd0c5%7C9274ee3f94254109a27f9fb15c10675d%7C0%7C0%7C637236034187789808&sdata=4f6m0myoo8%2FQiuSmJpSq96ybY-Dae62tGlAPtGGdi5g4%3D&reserved=0.
6. Wan TSK. Cancer cytogenetics: methodology revisited. Ann Lab Med 2014;34:413–25.
7. Speicher MR, Carter NP. The new cytogenetics: blurring the boundaries with molecular biology. Nat Rev Genet 2005;6:782–92.
8. Biegel JA. Cytogenetics and molecular genetics of childhood brain tumors. Neuro Oncol 2004;1:139–51.
9. Albertson DG, Collins C, McCormick F, et al. Chromosome aberrations in solid tumors. Nat Genet 2003;34:369–76.
10. Turner KM, Deshpande V, Beyter D, et al. Extrachromosomal Oncogene Amplification Drives Tumor Evolution and Genetic Heterogeneity. Nat Publ Gr 2017;543:122–5. Available at: https://nam03.safelinks.protection.outlook.com/?url=https%3A%2F%2Fpubmed.ncbi.nlm.nih.gov%2F28178237%2F&data=02%7C01%7CJ.Surendrakumar%40elsevier.com%7C3d2286b260054f383aac08-d7eacbd0c5%7C9274ee3f94254109a27f9fb15c10675d%7C0%7C0%7C637236034187789808&sdata=z1JhxXHgSviEbfkx8gr2%2BwvW9hOsq%2FVRYtzlrOCzfZE%3D&reserved=0.
11. Bielski CM, Zehir A, Penson AV, et al. Genome doubling shapes the evolution and prognosis of advanced cancers. Nat Genet 2018;50:1189–95.
12. Smith SC, Warren LM, Cooley LD. Maintaining a methods database to optimize solid tumor tissue culture: review of a 15-year database from a single institution. Cancer Genet 2019;233–234:96–101.
13. Horbinski C, Miller CR, Perry A. Gone FISHing: clinical lessons learned in brain tumor molecular diagnostics over the last decade. Brain Pathol 2011;21:57–73.

14. Park SH, Won J, Kim SI, et al. Molecular testing of brain tumor. J Pathol Transl Med 2017;51: 205–23.

15. Francis JM, Zhang CZ, Maire CL, et al. EGFR variant heterogeneity in glioblastoma resolved through single-nucleus sequencing. Cancer Discov 2014;4: 956–71.

16. Leeper HE, Caron AA, Decker PA, et al. IDH mutation, 1p19q codeletion and ATRX loss in WHO grade II gliomas. Oncotarget 2015;6:30295–305.

17. Suzuki H, Aoki K, Chiba K, et al. Mutational landscape and clonal architecture in grade II and III gliomas. Nat Genet 2015;47:458–68.

18. Buckner J, Giannini C, Eckel-Passow J, et al. Management of diffuse low-grade gliomas in adults–use of molecular diagnostics. Nat Rev Neurol 2017;13:340–51.

19. Dubuc AM, Ligon AH. From Prognostication to Personalized Medicine: Classification of Tumors of the Central Nervous System (CNS) Using Chromosomal Microarrays. Curr Genet Med Rep 2017;5: 117–24.

20. Neill SG, Hauenstein J, Li MM, et al. Copy number assessment in the genomic analysis of CNS neoplasia: an evidence-based review from the Cancer Genomics Consortium (CGC) Working Group on Primary CNS Tumors. Cancer Genet 2020. https://doi.org/10.1016/j.cancergen.2020.02.004.

21. Davare MA, Henderson JJ, Agarwal A, et al. Rare but recurrent ROS1 fusions resulting from chromosome 6q22 microdeletions are targetable oncogenes in glioma. Clin Cancer Res 2018;24:6471–82.

22. Kiehna EN, Arnush MR, Tamrazi B, et al. Novel GOPC(FIG)-ROS1 fusion in a pediatric high-grade glioma survivor. J Neurosurg Pediatr 2017; 20:51–5.

23. Mikhail FM, Biegel JA, Cooley LD, et al. Technical laboratory standards for interpretation and reporting of acquired copy-number abnormalities and copy-neutral loss of heterozygosity in neoplastic disorders: a joint consensus recommendation from the American College of Medical Genetics and Genomics (ACMG) and the Cancer Genomics Consortium (CGC). Genet Med 2019;21:1903–15.

24. Shendure J, Balasubramanian S, Church GM, et al. DNA sequencing at 40: past, present and future. Nature 2017;550:345–53.

25. Rizzo JM, Buck MJ. Key principles and clinical applications of "next-generation" DNA sequencing. Cancer Prev Res (Phila) 2012;5:887–900.

26. Le DT, Uram JN, Wang H, et al. PD-1 blockade in tumors with mismatch-repair deficiency. N Engl J Med 2015;372(26):2509–20.

27. Campbell BB, Light N, Fabrizio D, et al. Comprehensive analysis of hypermutation in human cancer. Cell 2017;171(5):1042–56.

28. Kerkhof J, Schenkel LC, Reilly J, et al. Clinical validation of copy number variant detection from targeted next-generation sequencing panels. J Mol Diagn 2017;19(6):905–20.

29. Capper D, Jones DTW, Sill M, et al. DNA methylation-based classification of central nervous system tumours. Nature 2018;555:469–74.

30. Jaunmuktane Z, Capper D, Jones DTW, et al. Methylation array profiling of adult brain tumours: diagnostic outcomes in a large, single centre. Acta Neuropathol Commun 2019;7:24.

31. Hovestadt V, Remke M, Kool M, et al. Robust molecular subgrouping and copy-number profiling of medulloblastoma from small amounts of archival tumour material using high-density DNA methylation arrays. Acta Neuropathol 2013;125:913–6.

Unsupervised Machine Learning in Pathology
The Next Frontier

Adil Roohi, BSc[a,b,1], Kevin Faust[b,c,1], Ugljesa Djuric, PhD[d], Phedias Diamandis, MD, PhD[d,e,f],*

KEYWORDS

• Pathology • Artificial intelligence • Deep learning • Unsupervised learning • Machine learning • Neuropathology

---

Key points

- Artificial intelligence and deep learning are increasingly prevalent in pathology and used to process large amounts of data.
- Unsupervised learning allows computational networks to discover patterns in data without significant training.
- This emerging type of machine learning facilitates a more human-like analytical approach, allowing for nuanced conclusions to be made without the need for specific pre-defined direction.

ABSTRACT

Applications of artificial intelligence and particularly deep learning to aid pathologists in carrying out laborious and qualitative tasks in histopathologic image analysis have now become ubiquitous. We introduce and illustrate how unsupervised machine learning workflows can be deployed in existing pathology workflows to begin learning autonomously through exploration and without the need for extensive direction. Although still in its infancy, this type of machine learning, which more closely mirrors human intelligence, stands to add another exciting layer of innovation to computational pathology and accelerate the transition to autonomous pathologic tissue analysis.

Non-standard abbreviations	
CNN	Convolutional neural network
TGCA	The Cancer Genome Atlas
t-SNE	t-Distributed Stochastic Neighbor Embedding
WHO	World Health Organization

Most of human and animal learning is unsupervised. If intelligence was a cake, unsupervised learning would be the cake and supervised learning would be the icing on the cake.
—Yann LeCun, Deep Learning Pioneer

---

[a] Harvard Extension School, 51 Brattle Street, Cambridge, MA 02138, USA; [b] Princess Margaret Cancer Centre, 101 College Street, Toronto, Ontario M5G 1L7, Canada; [c] Department of Computer Science, University of Toronto, 40 St. George Street, Toronto, Ontario M5S 2E4, Canada; [d] Laboratory Medicine Program, University Health Network, 200 Elizabeth Street, Toronto, Ontario M5G 2C4, Canada; [e] Department of Laboratory Medicine and Pathobiology, University of Toronto, Toronto, Ontario M5S 1A8, Canada; [f] Department of Medical Biophysics, University of Toronto, Toronto, Ontario, Canada
[1] Equal contribution.
* Corresponding author. Laboratory Medicine Program, University Health Network, 200 Elizabeth Street, Toronto, Ontario M5G 2C4, Canada.
E-mail address: p.diamandis@mail.utoronto.ca

Surgical Pathology 13 (2020) 349–358
https://doi.org/10.1016/j.path.2020.01.002

THE NEED FOR ARTIFICIAL AGENTS TO ANALYZE MEDICAL IMAGING DATA

There is a growing appreciation for the need to accelerate the transition of microscopic tissue analysis from one centered around glass slides, toward a more digital, automated, and quantitative discipline.[1,2] Even though this evolution has been met with both fear and excitement by pathologists, the adoption of machine learning is a trend that stretches far beyond pathology and is rather becoming a common theme across all of health care and society.[3,4] This revolution is perhaps partly driven by transformative changes in the ability to generate, digitally store, and process data. The cost of digital storage, for example, has decreased by almost 6 orders of magnitude over the past 4 decades, making it less of a barrier for data collection. This has been especially true for domains like pathology, where file sizes have been comparatively large with single glass slides often requiring a gigabyte of data for digital storage.

Regardless of the underlying reasons for this exponential decrease in the cost of data storage, these types of innovations are already changing how we use medical infrastructure and resources. For example, these technological improvements have led to the increasing reliance on advanced medical imaging (eg, computed tomography, MRIs) over the past 40 years and will likely continue to do so for the foreseeable future. As the medical community's ability to generate and store high-quality data continues to grow, the demand for highly specialized humans (pathologists and radiologists) needed to interpret the data will likely not be able to keep up. Specifically, this is becoming a reality in pathology, as the discipline's ability to digitally scan and store whole slide images at qualities suitable for diagnostic practice is also rapidly growing.[5] Moreover, the concurrent advent of artificial intelligence and deep learning could transform how histologic data are analyzed and used from each patient's specimen.[6,7]

THE PERILS AND PROMISES OF DEEP LEARNING FOR PATHOLOGIC IMAGE ANALYSIS

Although pattern recognition can be said to be an innate skill for the human brain, it is common practice to convert this diagnostic "art" into a set of teachable, highly reproducible, and objective set of rules to improve consistency among observers. This strategy has been particularly important for high-stakes decision in areas like medicine. For example, in pathology, trainees are encouraged to arrive at diagnoses by making a set of progressive decisions geared at carefully narrowing the differential diagnosis to a single or small set of likely diseases (eg, lesion vs no lesion; infectious vs neoplastic process). Development of such sets of reliable rules and robust decision tree-type frameworks not only improves reproducibility among humans but has also made this process highly conducive to automation by machines.

For example, in traditional machine learning approaches, computer engineers leverage these rules and frameworks to develop surrogate hand-crafted computer features that attempt to mimic or parallel the morphologic features (eg, necrosis, mitoses) that pathologists use to arrive to a diagnosis. Once digitized, the quantitative value of these multiple features can serve as objective morphologic signatures for image classification. Although these have been quite effective,[7] one limitation of this traditional approach is that the relatively small number of manually engineered patterns (100–1000s), are often unable to capture complex positional information that humans innately use to carry out specialized pattern recognition tasks. Recently however, transformative innovations in computer vision, particularly a form of artificial intelligence (AI) known as deep learning, has helped overcome this.[8] Particularly, a specific type of deep learning algorithm, known as convolutional neural networks (CNN), attempts to mimic how the human brain processes visual information and has allowed scientists to transition away from these laborious manual hand crafted features and instead rely on data to drive feature design.[9] Like the brain's visual cortex, the multilayered CNN architecture first detects elementary features (eg, color, shapes, edges) within an image and sequentially aggregates different combinations of the patterns to generate millions of advanced spatially dependant features of higher classification value.[8] Importantly, these features are computationally designed and selected and not reliant on humans for their generation. Once these features are developed and trained on a particular task, test images can be introduced to these networks to quantify the presence of these complex features and then use them to carry out classification tasks. With sufficient data and processing power that has recently become available, these novel computational tools were theoretically predicted to surpass the performance of traditional tools for classification.

This hypothesis was ultimately proven to be correct during the 2012 ImageNet computer vision competition.[10,11] Here, computer scientists annually compete to determine the most effective approaches and algorithms for classifying images that span 1000 different classes of common objects (eg, cats, dogs, planes). When this competition first started, the ImageNet winners used algorithms that were designed around the traditional hand-crafted feature approaches. These approaches had classification error rates of approximately 27%; much higher than a human given this same task (~3% error) and perhaps too high for any practical application. In 2012 however, AI pioneer Geoffrey Hinton and his team introduced, the first CNN-based algorithm in this image recognition competition and substantially reduced the winning error rate to 16%.[10,11] Every year since, sequential modifications have improved on his innovation, with state-of-the-art CNNs now equaling, and even surpassing, humans at classifying the diverse image types found in this competition. Although an impressive feat, many critics have rightfully pointed out that this competition represents a highly controlled environment and task that does not fully capture the dynamic decision-making capabilities of human observers in the real-world environment.

In recent years, these breakthroughs in deep learning approaches to pattern recognition have infiltrated the medical field.[12–16] Numerous studies have now shown that deep learning can perform many visual diagnostic tasks at levels that match or even exceed human experts in both primary care settings and more definitive pathologic analyses.[12,15] These systems are so robust that the tools have largely now become democratized, allowing anyone with access to data to develop and use them without the need for significant training in the computer sciences. This has been particularly effective in pathology, where repetitive patterns can be used to generate massive datasets that the algorithms can use to learn and classify future images (**Fig. 1**). However, despite these heralded successes, many surveys across all fields (eg, medicine, finance) find that most implementations of AI initiatives are met with significant challenges and failure. Arguably, a major component of these failures is the current inability for supervised learning approaches to fully mimic the diverse complement of skills and inference capabilities of the human observer. In this perspective, we wish to introduce the concept of unsupervised learning and how it differs from the supervised tasks that have now become ubiquitous in histopathologic image analysis. We supplement some of these theoretic concepts with examples from our own work to illustrate how unsupervised deep learning approaches can be introduced into pathology workflows to overcome some of the existing barriers

we believe are preventing the deployment of AI in pathology.

UNSUPERVISED LEARNING

Unsupervised learning fundamentally differs from supervised learning because it does not rely on specific classification instructions. Instead, it relies on autonomously grouping objects through exploration and discovery of the underlying pattern and structures in data. As alluded to in the quote at the beginning of this piece, this approach is viewed as the primary way we as humans collect information and build knowledge about the world around us. Although this undirected approach may not afford unsupervised learning the ability to resolve the same level of detail for specific user-defined tasks, it provides a highly flexible approach to define patterns in data that do not need to be predicted or anticipated. Unsupervised learning also affords humans with the ability to handle unanticipated changes in conditions and extend knowledge outside the training parameters (**Fig. 2**). The regular implementation of such strategies into machine learning workflows could help broaden AI-workflow performances in a wider spectrum of scenarios without the constant and infeasible task of continual needing to update supervised training parameters as knowledge and diagnostic goals evolve.

To illustrate the differences between supervised and unsupervised learning, we consider both continuous and discrete outputs generated by both approaches (see **Fig. 2**). A classic supervised classification task that uses continuous data would involve investigating if the aggressiveness of meningiomas (or another tumor type) can be predicted as a continuous function of the Ki-67 index (regression analysis). Conversely, the World Health Organization (WHO) current grading system represents a more discrete supervised classification task in which the combined presence of specific features (eg, necrosis, nucleoli), at varying amounts, could be sufficient to warrant a specific WHO grades (I vs II). Although these techniques are highly effective, there could, of course, be other ways to better organize the patterns, combinations, and respective amounts of features, like mitoses and necrosis. Importantly, although some of these patterns may not correlate with a desired task (aggressiveness), reoccurring patterns may provide important insight and have other important implications to the underlying biology of these tumors and help guide more personalized therapies. These are the types of "serendipitous" or "anomalous" patterns that are

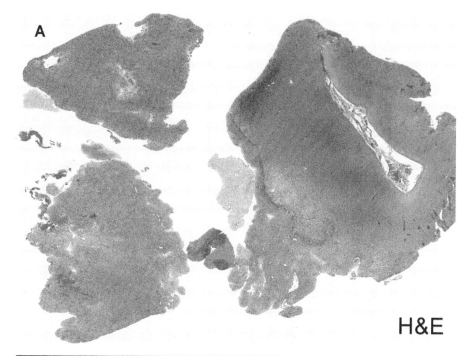

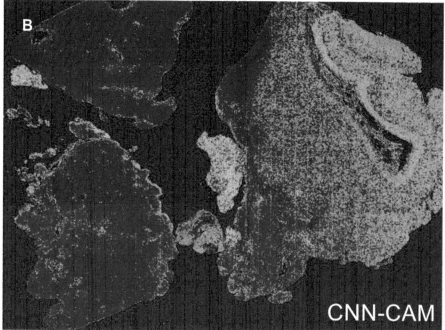

Blank Space: 29.92% (Black)
Grey Matter: 9.26% (Pink)
Meningioma: 0.51% (Brown)
Lymphoma: 1.29% (Brown)
Blood: 0.84% (Red)
Schwannoma: 0.32% (Brown)
Cerebellum: 0.10% (Pink)

White Matter: 0.61% (Pink)
Glioma: 52.83% (Brown)
Metastasis: 0.14% (Brown)
Necrosis: 3.92% (Light Pink)
Surgical: 0.09% (Magenta)
Dura: 0.18% (Dark Orchid)

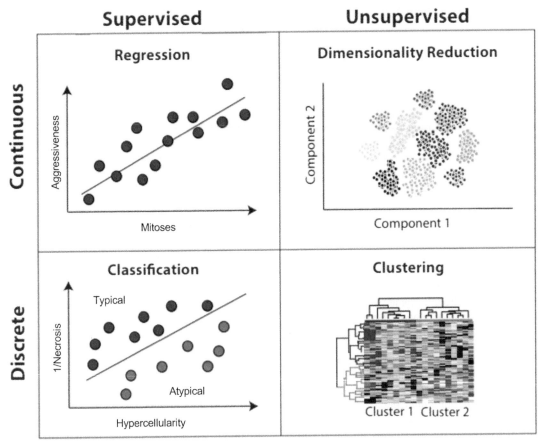

Fig. 2. Differences between machine learning methods. Illustrated are the distinct outputs of the 2 main groups of machine learning methods. In supervised learning, labeled samples with both input and output data are used to develop a model that can approximate the relationship between those values. The developed model can then be used to make future prediction of a specific output given a set of input values. In regression analysis, the output value is continuous, whereas for classic classification tasks, the output categorizes the test case into one specific class. In unsupervised learning, the algorithm uses only input data to propose the natural structure globally present within the data points, without the use of a specific output for guidance. Similar to supervised learning outputs, the outputs can be both continuous or grouped into more discrete clusters.

often discovered by expert pathologists who have seen high volumes of cases in their careers. Conversely, these are also the main types of patterns central to unsupervised analyses.

Dimensionality reduction techniques, such as principal component analysis, and t-SNE (t-distributed Stochastic Neighbor Embedding) provide data visualization outputs that allow

exploration into local and global patterns in continuous data. This information also can be discretized using hierarchical clustering, which facilitates the grouping of data into different clusters with an ontological tree highlighting the distance similarity of each data point to one another. Although these spatial and cluster associations are "unlabeled," they provide an initial starting point for the human

Fig. 1. Supervised annotation of a digital whole slide image using CNNs. (*A*) Hematoxylin-eosin (H&E)-stained digital slide image of an infiltrating glioblastoma showing the typical heterogeneous mixture of tumor, necrosis, brain tissue, and blood. (*B*) Corresponding CNN-generated class activation map (CAM) of the entire slide. The probability scores for each of the 13 trained classes of this CNN listed below the image provide a global overview of the tumor and tissue patterns detected. The most likely diagnosis of the lesion represented in this case based on these values is a glioma. Lesional areas are collectively depicted with a brown color on the CAM, whereas other tissue components are a different color. This depicts the powerful supervised capabilities of supervised classification tasks by CNN in pathology.

observer to find clinical or other relevant biological correlates that could explain why these associations arose. In this article, we provide some examples from our work to illustrate how we have used unsupervised approaches to help automate "anomaly" detection during routine classification tasks and also for automated ontological organization of tumor types without explicit instruction. Further development of such tools could serve to complement more supervised approaches by providing access to more advanced decision-making capabilities needed to better automate the diagnostic pathology workflow.

DIMENSIONALITY REDUCTION FOR HIGHLIGHTING ANOMALOUS CASES AND REDUCING ERRORS

Most current studies that use deep learning for computer vision in pathology involve highly focused and controlled classification tasks. Unfortunately, in the real world, there often can be extreme biological variability from case to case, even for common lesions like glioblastoma (eg, gliosarcomatous, small cell and epithelioid variants).[17] Similarly, tumor classification schemes are still evolving, making it cumbersome to continually tune and authoritatively validate complex machine learning classifiers.[18] As a result, unexpected classification errors can occur in these situations (eg, mistaking a small cell glioblastoma for a diffuse large B-cell lymphoma) or even when more elementary artifacts are encountered that were not comprehensively included in the training data. This includes differences in cellularity from edema, changes in the intensity of staining, and folds in tissue. In our hands, this phenomenon is perhaps one of the largest barriers to widespread adoption of these tools in pathology. Although this obstacle can theoretically be overcome with increasing amounts of data, the unpredictability of how tumor phenotypes and groupings will continue to change in the era of personalized medicine, where patients may receive a myriad of individualized therapies, can make such efforts extremely difficult to standardize (or "supervise").

To highlight how unsupervised learning approaches can help overcome these limitations, we recently explored how anomalies and artifacts can be effectively detected and flagged using the dimensionality reduction technique known as t-SNE.[19] Specifically, we generated approximately 80,000 training images spanning approximately 100 surgical cases to train and create a multiclass classifier that could annotate 13 common tissue classes encountered in neuropathology (eg, white

matter, dura, lymphoma, gliomas, blood, meningioma, metastasis) (see **Fig. 1**). When deploying our classifier in a traditional supervised manner to classify a set of 123 testing cases, it was able to correctly diagnose 86% of the test cases (14% errors). Interestingly, most errors arose from "untrained" and relatively "rare" tumor subtypes (eg, gliosarcoma, hemangioblastoma) that were not included in the original training set.

To address this issue, without having to develop additional training examples, we instead used unsupervised techniques to determine if outlier test cases could be efficiently detected as anomalous and prevent them from being classified incorrectly.[19] Toward this, we used the same CNN used to classify images shown in **Fig. 1**, to generate a t-SNE plot and visualize the learned representations within the network (**Fig. 3**). On this 2-dimensional (2D) grid, the proximity of 2 images (represented as individual dots) or groups of images (clusters of similarly colored dots) indicates their degree of similarity. Although the close proximity of the similarly colored dots represents the supervised component of learning, the distances between different classes is largely driven by unsupervised tissue patterns independently learned by the computer.

By closely examining the organization, many "intelligent" associations are evident. For example, the network grouped cellular tissue elements close together on the right half of the 2D plot. Similarly, the glioma image cluster (cluster of blue dots) is positionally closest to normal glial tissue (yellow/green/dark green dots), suggesting that the CNN could have learned some implicit patterns of similarities in these glial tissue elements. Moreover, more cohesive tumors (meningiomas, metastases) also appear close to one another on the plot (orange and purple dots). This organization of tissue classes demonstrates intelligible unsupervised learning that has been patterned within CNNs. From a practical perspective, this rich positional information on a plot can be used to automate the detection of anomalous cases into histopathologic image analysis. When a test image (a slide the computer has not seen before) is regionally sampled and overlaid onto these plots (depicted as red diamonds in **Fig. 3**), the overlap between test images and those found in the training set suggests high similarities in the tissue architecture (see **Fig. 3**A). However, when the CNN is presented with a previously unencountered class (eg, hemangioblastoma) or variant (eg, gliosarcoma), the vast differences in the histologic patterns (and imaging data structures) between the rare/untrained testing cases and stereotypical training datasets become

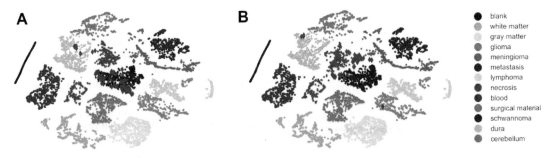

Fig. 3. Dimensionality reduction for anomaly detection. Planar representation of the internal high-dimensional data structure of the final layer of the 13-class CNN used to generate the CAM in **Fig. 1**. Each colored dot represents an ~512 μm^2 histologic image. During supervised training, images belonging to the same class allow the CNN to optimize features for robust classification. The t-SNE plot of these data allow us to understand the unsupervised association of the global data structure. In (*A*), images patched from a test image (red diamonds, glioblastoma) are overlaid onto the t-SNE plot. The overlap of the test and training images suggests that the data structure of the test image is similar to the training image. In (*B*), image patches from the test image of an untrained class (hemangioblastoma) show a distinct data structure compared with the training images. This suggests an anomalous or unlearned tissue class. (*Adapted from* Faust K, Xie Q, Han D, et al. Visualizing histopathologic deep learning classification and anomaly detection using nonlinear feature space dimensionality reduction. *BMC Bioinformatics*. 2018;19(1):173; with permission.)

immediately evident. These differences are depicted by the images grouping in a unique and nonoverlapping area of the t-SNE plot (see **Fig. 3B**). We leverage this property to objectively define untrained/anomalies in data and prevent classification errors in these challenging circumstances. In fact, even without any modifications to the network or use of additional data, we were able to reduce errors by more than 60% using this alternative approach.[19] As a result, unsupervised visualization of data structures provides immediately available approaches to monitor unexpected pathologies. This approach can potentially not only help reduce errors but also excitingly potentially detect common tumor with anomalous biology (ie, significant infiltration by lymphocytes) with important implications for emerging treatments, like immunotherapy.

CLUSTERING TO AUTOMATE ONTOLOGICAL ARRANGEMENT OF MICROSCOPIC PATTERNS ON A LARGE SCALE

Although the qualitative detection of novel/anomalous cases is an important component of the microscopic examination, the ability to link recurring patterns into potentially relevant subgroups also represents an advanced and important skill many pathologists contribute to the ontological organization of tumors through their diagnostic practice. Although the baseline tumor subtypes have already been largely defined, this skill will likely continue to help in characterizing new diseases, outbreaks, and

differential responses to emerging treatment regimens. This type of specialized pattern grouping task also can be mirrored using unsupervised clustering algorithms that ontologically arrange cases into discrete groups based on shared features.

To highlight how this tasked could be mirrored in silico, we recently also developed a 74-class tissue classifier mostly composed of tumors outlined in the WHO classification guide for brain tumors. This diagnostic manual, developed from input from many international experts, provides a consensus approach to how tumors should be organized based on their microscopic features, molecular characteristics, and understood biology (gliomas, meningiomas, with different subtypes within each class).[20] Notably, some microscopic features, like high nuclear-to-cytoplasmic ratio, can be shared between biologically unrelated classes. As such, this manual also provides guidelines to help the practicing pathologist avoid known diagnostic pitfalls and effectively exclude entities that exist on the differential diagnosis.

Toward potentially being able to automate such large-scale classification schemes, we recently used 1691 whole slide images to generate approximately 850,000 images spanning 74 different tissues classes to train a CNN.[21] By clustering the classes based on 512 high-level features optimized during the training of the neural network, we found that indeed the unsupervised hierarchical arrangement of classes, based solely on their histologic patterns, created a framework similar to that proposed in the WHO (**Fig. 4**). Importantly, these unsupervised approaches allow for examination of the individual features that the computer optimized and used to group the tumor classes. This exercise revealed the computer can autonomously optimize and use many of the same morphologic features (eg, perinuclear halos, mucin, epithelium, luminal structures) that pathologists use to guide grouping.[21] Interestingly, even "errors" appeared to be easily explainable. This included grouping of highly vascular tumors (eg, hemangioblastoma and angiomatous meningioma, see **Fig. 4**C) or lesions with a high nuclear-to-cytoplastic ratio (eg, glioblastoma and diffuse large B-cell lymphoma; see **Fig. 4**B). Together, this highlights the ability of unsupervised machine learning approaches to automate advanced organizational tasks and propose a complex grouping of histologic information without the need for direct instruction.

SUMMARY AND OUTLOOK

Although much of pathology can be taught through concrete knowledge and patterns described in textbooks, it is not uncommon for even seasoned pathologists to encounter lesions they have never previously seen. These could be due to extremely rare lesions that arise only a handful of times over a pathologist's career, newly emerging diseases (eg, microcephaly induced by Zika virus infection), changes to therapeutic management of common diseases, or even artifacts that arise during the slide preparation process. Although each of these may be rare events, serendipitous observations and a constant sense of uncertainty is a regular part of everyday pathologic analysis. As increasing amounts of data are generated in an era in which personalized therapies are on the horizon, these rare examples will likely increase in frequency and could provide clues to subgroups of patients who experience durable and exceptional

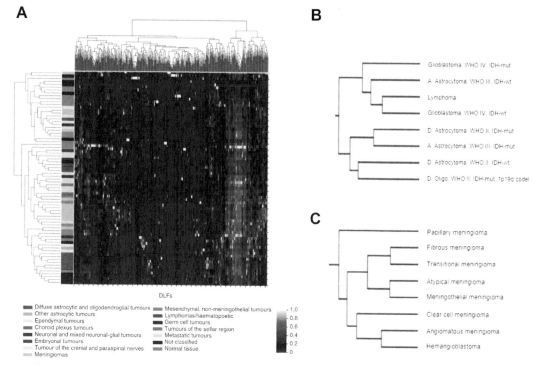

Fig. 4. Clustering for unsupervised ontological arrangement of morphologic patterns by deep learning. (*A*) Hierarchical arrangement of 74 trained classes (vertical axis) based on 512 deep learning derived features (DLF, horizontal axis). Many tumors belonging to the same board tumor class (eg, metastasis, diffuse gliomas, meningiomas) are grouped together. Other tumors were grouped based on overlapping morphologic features (mucin in chordoma and chondrosarcoma). (*B*) and (*C*) provide representative subtrees of the overall dendrogram, highlighting the unsupervised clustering/relationships detected between tumor subtypes based on the global patterns of deep learning feature activations. (*Adapted from* Faust K, Bala S, van Ommeren R, et al. Intelligent feature engineering and ontological mapping of brain tumour histomorphologies by deep learning. *Nat Mach Intell.* 2019;1(7):316-321; with permission.)

responses to treatment. AI will need to extend beyond traditional supervised approaches and develop more humanlike unsupervised approaches to pattern recognition in histologic image analysis to be a viable and useful tool for human pathologists.

In this article, we presented and discussed some of our own experiences with trying to overcome the challenges facing machine learning by shifting toward more unsupervised learning techniques and outputs. Although there could be concerns that these tools will lead to the eventual replacement of human pathologists, we hope the provided examples highlight that even after these "intelligent" outputs are generated, these automated observations require significant human insights to properly vet the findings in the context of other molecular and clinical information. In an era in which digital data continue to grow at an exponential rate, it is likely that these tools will serve to augment the productivity of pathologists and allow them to serve more important integrative roles in both the clinical and investigational components of their profession.

AUTHOR CONTRIBUTIONS

All authors contributed to the article equally.

ACKNOWLEDGMENTS

Funding support for the Diamandis Lab and trainees is provided by the Princess Margaret Cancer Foundation, University of Toronto's Department of Laboratory Medicine and Pathobiology, American Society of Clinical Oncology Career Development Award (ASCO-CDA), and The Brain Tumour Charity Expanding Theories Research Grant (GN-000560). U. Djuric is supported through a University of Toronto Department of Laboratory Medicine and Pathobiology research fellowship award. The authors thank Ms Clare Fiala for constructive feedback.

COMPETING INTERESTS

The authors declare no conflicts of interest.

REFERENCES

1. Djuric U, Zadeh G, Aldape K, et al. Precision histology: how deep learning is poised to revitalize histomorphology for personalized cancer care. NPJ Precis Oncol 2017;1. https://doi.org/10.1038/s41698-017-0022-1.
2. Jha S, Topol EJ, K.C., et al. Adapting to artificial intelligence. JAMA 2016;316(22):2353.
3. Sarwar S, Dent A, Faust K, et al. Physician perspectives on integration of artificial intelligence into diagnostic pathology. NPJ Digit Med 2019;2(1):28.
4. Lakhani P, Sundaram B. Deep learning at chest radiography: automated classification of pulmonary tuberculosis by using convolutional neural networks. Radiology 2017;284(2):574–82.
5. Campanella G, Hanna MG, Geneslaw L, et al. Clinical-grade computational pathology using weakly supervised deep learning on whole slide images. Nat Med 2019;25(8):1301–9.
6. Coudray N, Ocampo PS, Sakellaropoulos T, et al. Classification and mutation prediction from non-small cell lung cancer histopathology images using deep learning. Nat Med 2018;24(10):1559–67.
7. Yu K-H, Zhang C, Berry GJ, et al. Predicting non-small cell lung cancer prognosis by fully automated microscopic pathology image features. Nat Commun 2016;7:12474.
8. LeCun Y, Bengio Y, Hinton G. Deep learning. Nature 2015;521(7553):436–44.
9. Madabhushi A, Lee G. Image analysis and machine learning in digital pathology: challenges and opportunities. Med Image Anal 2016;33:170–5.
10. Simonyan K, Zisserman A. Very deep convolutional networks for large-scale image recognition. 2014. Available at: https://scholar.google.com/scholar?q=Very%20Deep%20Convolutional%20Networks%20for%20Large-Scale%20Image%20Recognition.%20arXiv%202015.
11. Deng J, Dong W, Socher R, et al. ImageNet: A Large-Scale Hierarchical Image Database. Available at: http://www.image-net.org/papers/imagenet_cvpr09.pdf. Accessed December 30, 2017.
12. Mobadersany P, Yousefi S, Amgad M, et al. Predicting cancer outcomes from histology and genomics using convolutional networks. Proc Natl Acad Sci U S A 2018;115(13):E2970–9.
13. Ebert LC, Heimer J, Schweitzer W, et al. Automatic detection of hemorrhagic pericardial effusion on PMCT using deep learning - a feasibility study. Forensic Sci Med Pathol 2017;13(4):426–31.
14. Esteva A, Kuprel B, Novoa RA, et al. Dermatologist-level classification of skin cancer with deep neural networks. Nature 2017;542(7639):115–8.
15. Xie Q, Faust K, Van Ommeren R, et al. Deep learning for image analysis: personalizing medicine closer to the point of care. Crit Rev Clin Lab Sci 2019;56(1):61–73.
16. Litjens G, Sánchez CI, Timofeeva N, et al. Deep learning as a tool for increased accuracy and efficiency of histopathological diagnosis. Sci Rep 2016;6(1):26286.

17. Diamandis P, Aldape KD. Insights from molecular profiling of adult glioma. J Clin Oncol 2017;35(21):2386–93.

18. Diamandis P, Aldape K. World Health Organization 2016 classification of central nervous system tumors. Neurol Clin 2018;36(3):439–47.

19. Faust K, Xie Q, Han D, et al. Visualizing histopathologic deep learning classification and anomaly detection using nonlinear feature space dimensionality reduction. BMC Bioinformatics 2018;19(1):173.

20. Louis DN, Perry A, Reifenberger G, et al. The 2016 World Health Organization Classification of Tumors of the Central Nervous System: a summary. Acta Neuropathol 2016;131(6). https://doi.org/10.1007/s00401-016-1545-1.

21. Faust K, Bala S, van Ommeren R, et al. Intelligent feature engineering and ontological mapping of brain tumour histomorphologies by deep learning. Nat Mach Intell 2019;1(7):316–21.

Printed and bound by CPI Group (UK) Ltd, Croydon, CR0 4YY

03/10/2024

01040372-0012